Diabetic Cooking

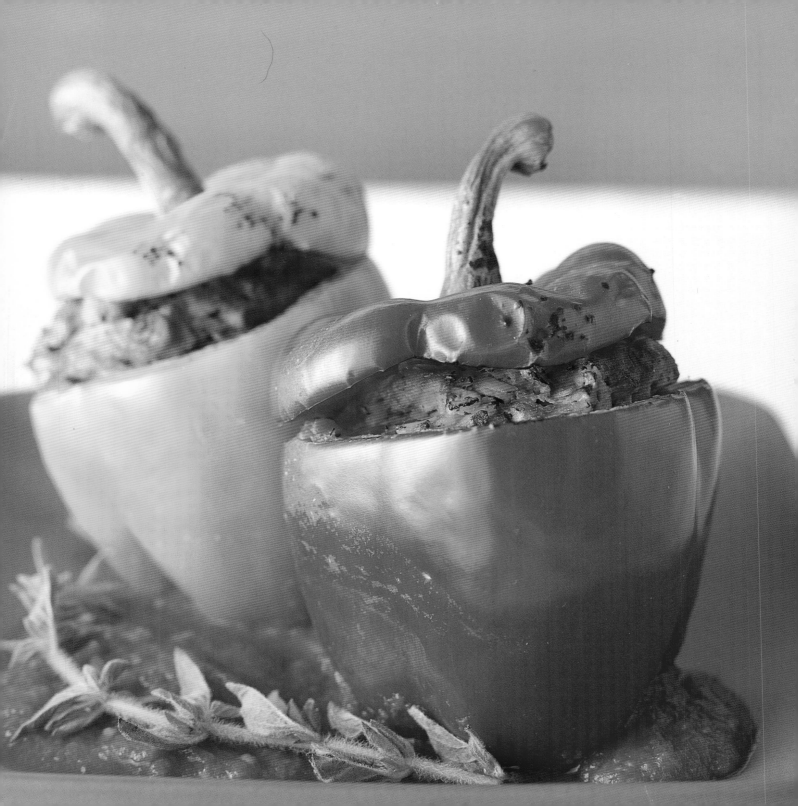

Diabetic Cooking

By Mary Jane Finsand & Karin Cadwell, Ph.D., R.N.

STERLING
INNOVATION
A Division of Sterling Publishing Co., Inc.
New York

Library of Congress Cataloging-in-Publication Data Available

2 4 6 8 10 9 7 5 3 1

Published in 2007 by Sterling Publishing Co., Inc.
387 Park Avenue South, New York NY 10016
This book was originally published as *Quick Cooks' Kitchen: Diabetic Recipes* and is comprised of material
from the following Sterling titles that have been revised and updated by Karin Cadwell:
The Diabetic High Fiber Cookbook © 1985 by Mary Jane Finsand
The Complete Diabetic Cookbook © 1987 by Sterling Publishing Co., Inc.
Diabetic Snack & Appetizer Cookbook © 1987 by Mary Jane Finsand
Diabetic Sweet Tooth Cookbook © 1993 by Mary Jane Finsand
Great International Diabetic Desserts © 1999 by Karin Cadwell
Quick & Delicious Diabetic Desserts © 1992 by Mary Jane Finsand
Diabetic Cookies © 1994 by Mary Jane Finsand
Great Diabetic Desserts & Sweets © 1995 by Karin Cadwell and Edith White
Diabetic Sweet Treats © 1997 by Karin Cadwell
The Diabetic Chocolate Cookbook © 1984 by Mary Jane Finsand

© 2005 by Sterling Publishing Co., Inc.
Photographs © 2005 by Theresa Raffetto
Distributed in Canada by Sterling Publishing
c/o Canadian Manda Group, 165 Dufferin Street
Toronto, Ontario, Canada M6K 3H6
Distributed in the United Kingdom by GMC Distribution Services
Castle Place, 166 High Street, Lewes, East Sussex, England BN7 1XU
Distributed in Australia by Capricorn Link (Australia) Pty. Ltd.
P.O. Box 704, Windsor, NSW 2756, Australia

Design by Liz Trovato
Photographs by Theresa Raffetto
Food Stylist: Victoria Granof
Prop Stylist: Sharon Ryan

Printed in China
All rights reserved

Sterling ISBN-13: 978-1-4027-4351-1
ISBN-10: 1-4027-4351-3

For information about custom editions, special sales, premium and
corporate purchases, please contact Sterling Special Sales
Department at 800-805-5489 or specialsales@sterlingpub.com.

Contents

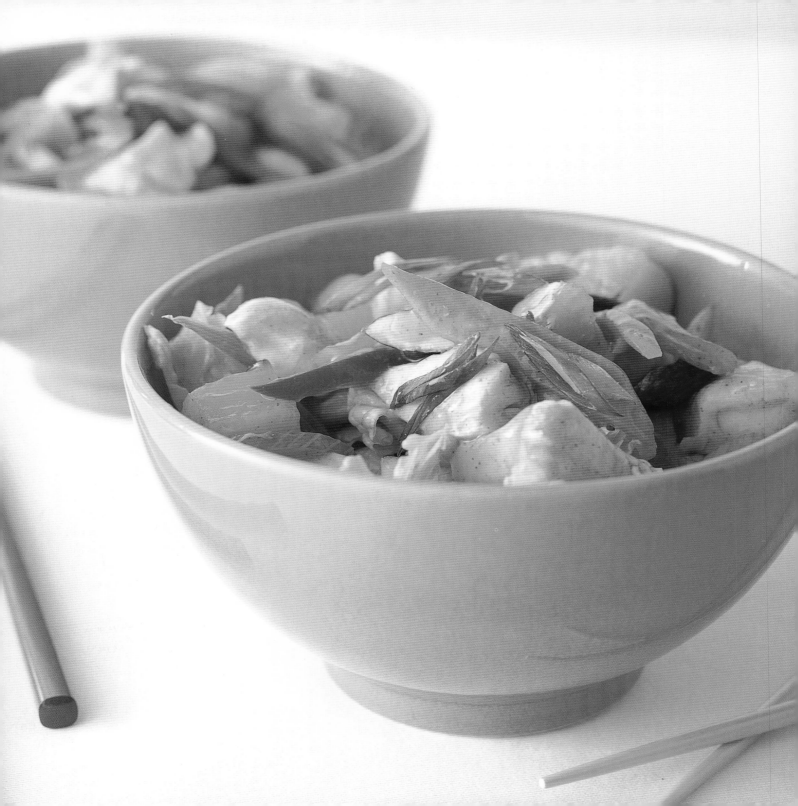

Introduction

With so many options for a quick meal these days—quality frozen, prepped, and ready-to-heat foods; take-out and delivery; and microwavable everything—there seems to be little reason to cook! In addition, nearly all these options are offered with a diabetic-friendly hook. So, if you need a quick meal and you are watching your blood-glucose level, you may still ask—why turn on your stove at all? *Diabetic Cooking* provides you with over 240 recipes full of home-cooked goodness that satisfy the busy chef in us all.

When you think of comfort foods and home-style cooking, you usually don't think many of these sweets and savories fall within the diabetic guidelines. The recipes here, however, will help you create more tasteful and varied meals, while reducing and simplifying the day-to-day preparation of healthful, good food. By using the simple exchange values (for exchange lists from the American Diabetes Association, see pages 213–219), you can whip up a gourmet meal in no time and without fear of overindulgence.

Prolonging life and controlling diabetes are essential factors in the consideration of a diet plan. Even if you do not have diabetes, you should be aware of your total calorie intake and compare it to your total calorie output daily. To make weight reduction or a healthy diet as pleasant and easy as possible, it is important to realize that eating and preparing the food can still be made an enjoyable experience, even for a novice chef.

In this cookbook you will find recipes from a variety of cuisines—some have international origins and some are decidedly domestic. All, however, are diabetic-friendly and will satiate your hunger but not leave you feeling deprived of certain foods. The portion sizes and serving suggestions try to help us home cooks achieve realistic goals toward moderation in our diets. You get nutritional balance, great flavors, and recipes that will get meals on the table with speed and ease.

Cooks' Tips

Here is some general advice to always consider when you are in the kitchen:

- Always read the recipe from start to finish before beginning your prep. Make sure you understand the directions and reread anything that seems unclear to you.

- Serving sizes vary throughout the book, ranging from single servings up to 16 or more in some cases. Carefully check each recipe and simply multiply or divide the ingredient amounts to suit your needs.

- Start by getting all your ingredients within reach and do all your prep work before beginning to cook.

That way, you can cruise through the instructions without any problems.

Basic Tools

You can create any of the recipes in this book with just a few basic kitchen tools:

Cutting board: At least one board in either wood or plastic is a must-have. Whichever you choose, be sure to get one that is large enough for unhindered chopping and small enough for easy washing by hand or in the dishwasher. For food safety, remember to use separate boards (or separate sides of one board) for cutting produce and raw meats and to wash the boards thoroughly between uses.

Chef's knife: Select a top-quality knife and keep it sharp for optimum performance. This knife comes in 6-, 8-, 10-, and 12-inch lengths. The 8-inch one gets our vote for versatility. It lets you cut meats, chop vegetables, and mince garlic and herbs in no time flat.

Paring knife: A paring knife usually comes with a 3- or 4-inch blade and makes short work of trimming mushrooms, peeling fruits, and other similar tasks.

Vegetable peeler: This tool is ideal for peeling thin-skinned root vegetables such as carrots, potatoes, parsnips, cucumbers, and even young butternut squash. Be sure to get a peeler with a swivel blade and a comfortable handle.

Measuring cups and spoons: Get a nested set of dry measuring cups for measuring rice, pasta, beans, and frozen peas and corn. Use a liquid measure for broth, tomatoes, and other liquid ingredients. The same set of nested spoons can be used for dry and wet items.

Wooden spoons: Wooden spoons are good for most mixing and stirring tasks. They don't scratch pots, pans, and dishes, and their shallow bowls are perfectly suited for stirring. Their handles stay cool, and they don't melt if you accidentally leave them touching a hot pot.

Large metal spoons: A good-size spoon with a deep bowl is ideal for stirring chunky, hearty soups and sauces.

Ladle: A ladle with a half-cup capacity is great for serving chowders and lighter-based soups.

Saucepans and pots: The smaller of the two has one handle and is called a saucepan; the larger has two handles and is called a pot. Make sure you get a snug fitting lid for whatever you have. The pot itself should be heavy and a nonstick interior is not necessary.

When choosing casseroles or baking dishes, the heaviest is usually the best. The heaviest-gauge pans spread and hold the heat evenly, thereby cooking the contents evenly. Lids with casseroles are very helpful. Glass casseroles or baking dishes may be covered with aluminum foil for the oven and plastic wrap for the refrigerator, but lids are prefered with other materials.

Casserole Containers
  7 x 11 x 2 yields 6 to 8 cups
  9 x 9 x 2 yields 10 cups
  9 x 13 x 2 yields 15 cups

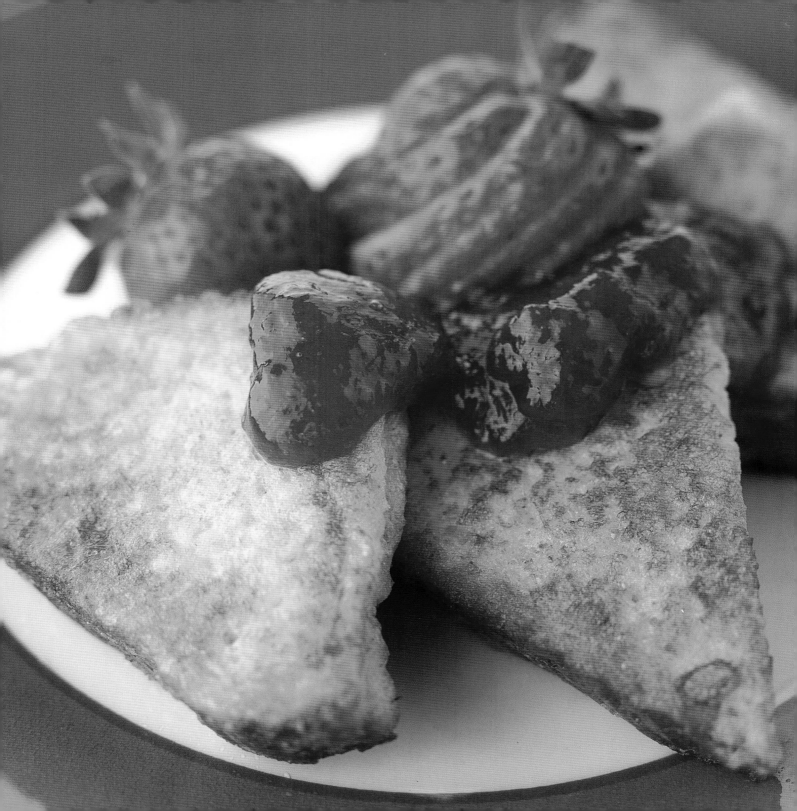

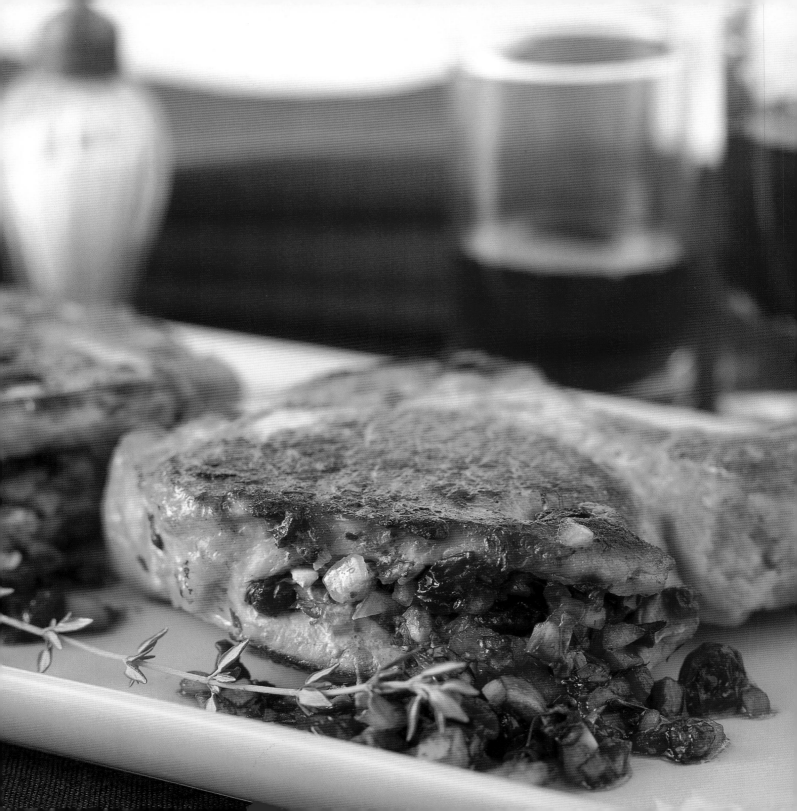

Metric Equivalents

The recipes that appear in this cookbook use the standard United States method for measuring liquid and dry or solid ingredients (teaspoons, tablespoons, and cups). The information on this chart is provided to help cooks outside the U.S. successfully use these recipes. All equivalents are approximate.

Metric Equivalents for Different Types of Ingredients

A standard cup measure of a dry or solid ingredient will vary in weight depending on the type of ingredient. A standard cup of liquid is the same volume for any type of liquid. Use the following chart when converting standard cup measures to grams (weight) or milliliters (volume).

Standard Cup	Fine Powder (e.g. flour)	Grain (e.g. rice)	Granular (e.g. sugar)	Liquid Solids (e.g. butter)	Liquid (e.g. milk)
1	140 g	150 g	190 g	200 g	240 ml
$3/4$	105 g	113 g	143 g	150 g	180 ml
$2/3$	93 g	100 g	125 g	133 g	160 ml
$1/2$	70 g	75 g	95 g	100 g	120 ml
$1/3$	47 g	50 g	63 g	67 g	80 ml
$1/4$	35 g	38 g	48 g	50 g	60 ml
$1/8$	18 g	19 g	24 g	25 g	30 ml

Useful Equivalents for Liquid Ingredients by Volume

$1/4$ tsp =				1 ml
$1/2$ tsp =				2 ml
1 tsp =				5 ml
3 tsp =	1 tbls =		$1/2$ fl oz =	15 ml
	2 tbls =	$1/8$ cup =	1 fl oz =	30 ml
	4 tbls =	$1/4$ cup =	2 fl oz =	60 ml
	$5^1/3$ tbls =	$1/3$ cup =	3 fl oz =	80 ml
	8 tbls =	$1/2$ cup =	4 fl oz =	120 ml
	$10^2/3$ tbls =	$2/3$ cup =	5 fl oz =	160 ml
	12 tbls =	$3/4$ cup =	6 fl oz =	180 ml
	16 tbls =	1 cup =	8 fl oz =	240 ml
	1 pt =	2 cups =	16 fl oz =	480 ml
	1 qt =	4 cups =	32 fl oz =	960 ml
			33 fl oz =	1000 ml = 1 l

Useful Equivalents for Dry Ingredients by Weight

(To convert ounces to grams, multiply the number of ounces by 30.)

1 oz	=	$1/16$ lb	=	30 g
4 oz	=	$1/4$ lb	=	120 g
8 oz	=	$1/2$ lb	=	240 g
12 oz	=	$3/4$ lb	=	360 g
16 oz	=	1 lb	=	480 g

Useful Equivalents for Length

(To convert inches to centimeters, multiply the number of inches by 2.5.)

1 in =				2.5 cm
6 in =	$1/2$ ft =			15 cm
12 in =	1 ft =			30 cm
36 in =	3 ft =	1 yd =		90 cm
40 in =				100 cm = 1 m

Useful Equivalents for Cooking/Oven Temperatures

	Fahrenheit	Celsius	Gas Mark
Freeze Water	32° F	0° C	
Room Temperature	68° F	20° C	
Boil Water	212° F	100° C	
Bake	325° F	160° C	3
	350° F	180° C	4
	375° F	190° C	5
	400° F	200° C	6
	425° F	220° C	7
	450° F	230° C	8
Broil			Grill

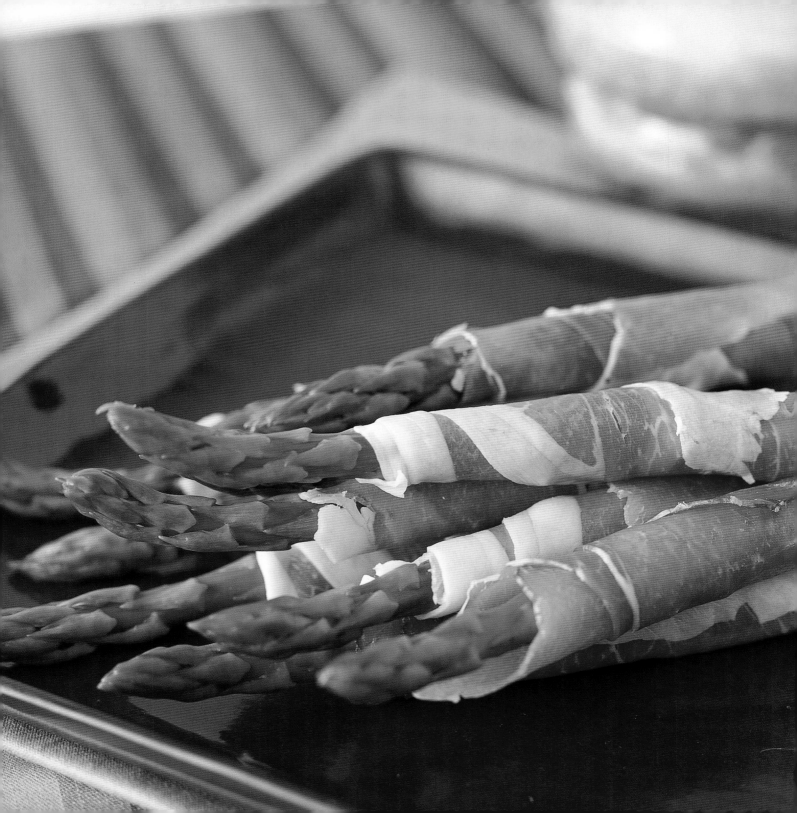

Appetizers

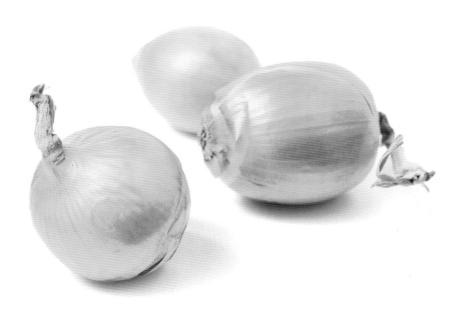

Appetizer Meatballs

MAKES 75 BALLS (15 SERVINGS)

3/4 *pound ground beef*

1/4 *pound ground pork*

3/4 *cup 4-grain cereal*

1/4 *cup water chestnuts, finely chopped*

1/4 *teaspoon Worcestershire sauce*

1/2 *cup skim milk*

1/2 *teaspoon garlic salt*

few drops Tabasco sauce

● Combine all ingredients and mix well. Shape into 75 small balls. In a nonstick pan, brown well over low heat. Place in chafing dish; add 1/2 cup warm water. Use toothpicks to serve.

EACH SERVING: ABOUT 114 CALORIES, 6 G PROTEIN, 6 G CARBOHYDRATE, 7 G TOTAL FAT (3 G SATURATED), 23 MG CHOLESTEROL, 84 MG SODIUM. EXCHANGE, EACH SERVING: 1 MEDIUM-FAT MEAT

Onion Dip

MAKES 3/4 CUP

4 *ounces plain low-calorie yogurt*

1/4 *cup onions, finely chopped*

1 *teaspoon lemon juice*

1 *tablespoon parsley*

dash hot pepper sauce

dash horseradish

salt and pepper to taste

● Combine all ingredients. Chill thoroughly.

ABOUT 89 CALORIES, 7 G PROTEIN, 12 G CARBOHYDRATE, 2 G TOTAL FAT (1 G SATURATED), 7 MG CHOLESTEROL, 83 MG SODIUM. EXCHANGE: 1/2 MILK, 1/2 VEGETABLE

Onion Dip

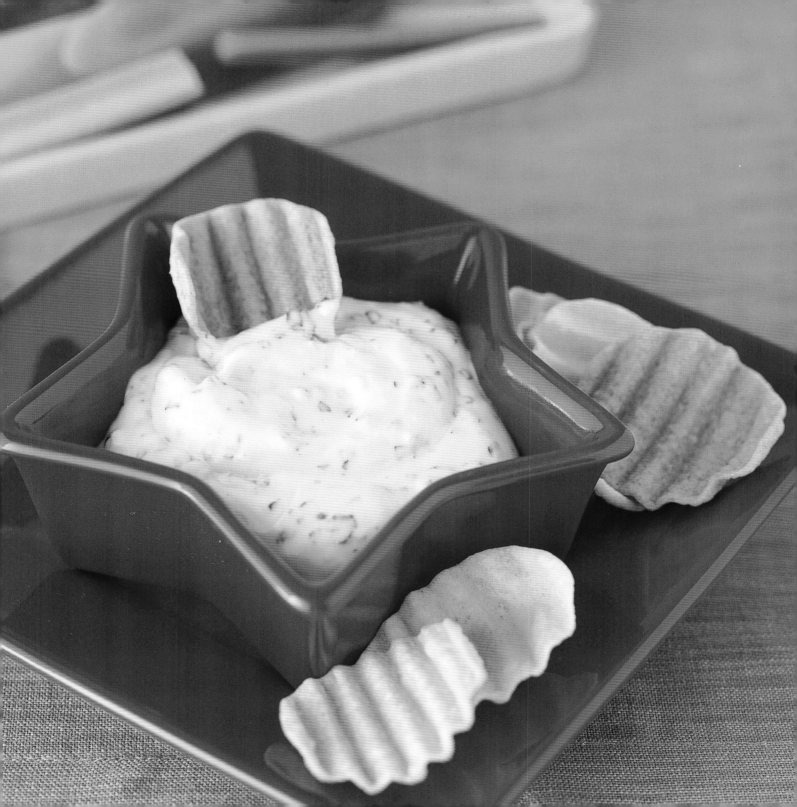

PREP TIME: 20 MINUTES   COOK TIME: 30 MINUTES

Super Nachos

MAKES 8 SERVINGS

8 ounces firm tofu (bean curd), drained and cut
  into 1-inch cubes

1 1/2 cups water

1 1/4 cups onion, chopped

2 cloves garlic, minced

3/4 cup pasta sauce

dash Tabasco sauce

6 ounces ground beef

1/2 cup mushrooms, chopped

2 teaspoons chili powder

1 teaspoon paprika

1/2 teaspoon ground cumin

1/2 teaspoon oregano

1 teaspoon no-salt seasoning

4 corn tortillas

4 ounces Cheddar cheese, grated

4 cups lettuce, shredded

2 cups tomatoes, diced

1 cup red pepper, chopped

2 cups green pepper, chopped

picante sauce

● In a small saucepan, combine tofu, 1 cup of the water, 2 tablespoons of the chopped onion, and garlic. Bring to a boil. Reduce heat and simmer 10 minutes. Drain off the water. Put the mixture in a food processor. Add pasta sauce and process until smooth. Season with Tabasco sauce. Set aside.

● Meanwhile, brown meat with chopped mushrooms and 1 tablespoon of the chopped onions. Add seasonings and remaining water and simmer for 10 minutes or until water evaporates. On baking sheet, arrange tortillas in a single layer. Bake at 450°F until crisp, about 4 minutes on each side. Preheat broiler. Spread on each tortilla 1/4 of the tofu mixture, then 1/4 of the seasoned beef, then 1/4 of the grated cheese. Broil until cheese is bubbly, about 5 minutes. Place each tortilla on a separate plate. Surround each tortilla with 1/4 of each vegetable—lettuce, tomatoes, onions, and red and green pepper. Serve picante sauce on the side.

EACH SERVING: ABOUT 174 CALORIES, 12 G PROTEIN, 17 G CARBOHYDRATE,
8 G TOTAL FAT (3 G SATURATED), 19 MG CHOLESTEROL, 278 MG SODIUM.
EXCHANGE, EACH SERVING: 1 BREAD, 1 HIGH-FAT MEAT

Sesame Cheese Balls

MAKES 20 BALLS

1 3-ounce package cream cheese, softened
1/4 cup blue cheese
1/4 cup dried beef, minced
dash cayenne pepper
1/4 cup sesame seeds, toasted

● Blend cheeses with dried beef and cayenne pepper. Shape into 20 small balls. Chill. Roll in sesame seeds.

EACH BALL: ABOUT 25 CALORIES, 2 G PROTEIN, 1 G CARBOHYDRATE, 2 G
TOTAL FAT (1 G SATURATED), 3 MG CHOLESTEROL, 145 MG SODIUM.
EXCHANGE, EACH BALL: 1/2 FAT

Danish-Style Meatballs

MAKES 40 MEATBALLS

2 pounds lean ground round
1/2 pound lean ground pork
3/4 cup all-purpose flour
3/4 cup evaporated skim milk
3 eggs
2 onions, cut in pieces
2 teaspoons salt
1 teaspoon granulated sugar replacement
1/2 teaspoon ground ginger

● Combine ground round and ground pork in a large bowl. With a spoon or your hands, work until well mixed. Combine remaining ingredients in a food processor with a steel blade or in a blender. Blend until smooth. Pour into meats, and work until completely incorporated. Form into 40 small balls. Heat a large kettle half full of water to boiling. Drop meatballs individually into the boiling water. Do not crowd kettle. When meat is firm and brown, remove with a slotted spoon. To serve: Fry gently in a skillet over low heat until browned. You can make these meatballs any time and then freeze them in small amounts to be used later.

EACH MEATBALL: ABOUT 88 CALORIES, 6 G PROTEIN, 3 G CARBOHYDRATE,
5 G TOTAL FAT (2 G SATURATED), 37 MG CHOLESTEROL, 145 MG SODIUM.
EXCHANGE, EACH MEATBALL: 1 MEDIUM-FAT MEAT

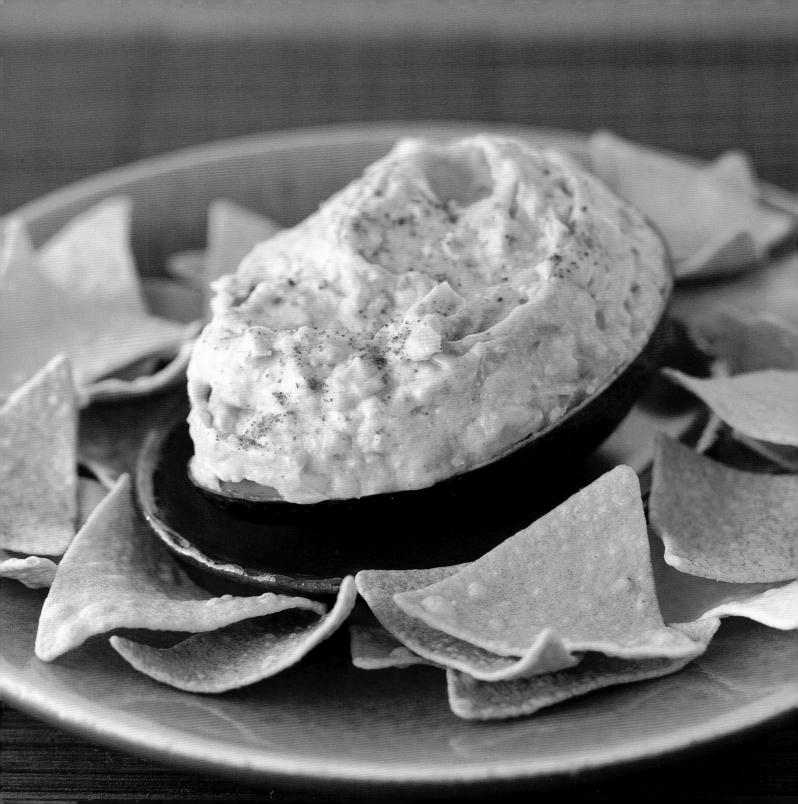

Avocado Crisps

MAKES 9 SERVINGS

1 very ripe avocado

1 teaspoon lemon juice

1 teaspoon grated onion

1 teaspoon onion salt

1 teaspoon paprika

1/2 teaspoon marjoram

thin crackers

● Peel and mash avocado. Add remaining ingredients. Beat until smooth. Spread thinly on crackers.

EACH SERVING: ABOUT 90 CALORIES, 2 G PROTEIN, 13 G CARBOHYDRATE, 4 G TOTAL FAT (TRACE SATURATED), 0 MG CHOLESTEROL, 280 MG SODIUM. EXCHANGE, EACH SERVING: 1 BREAD, 1 FAT

Cheese Wafers

MAKES 5 DOZEN WAFERS (20 SERVINGS)

3/4 cup all-purpose flour

dash cayenne pepper

1/4 cup sesame seeds, toasted

1/2 cup margarine, softened

2 cups sharp Cheddar cheese, shredded

1 cup bran cereal

● Stir together flour and pepper. Set aside. Measure sesame seeds into small shallow bowl. Beat margarine and cheese until very light and fluffy. Stir in the cereal. Add flour mixture, mixing until well combined. Drop by rounded teaspoonfuls into sesame seeds. Coat evenly. Place on ungreased baking sheets. Flatten with fork that has been dipped in flour. Bake at 350°F for 12 minutes or until lightly browned around edges. Remove immediately from baking sheets. Cool on wire racks.

EACH SERVING: ABOUT 100 CALORIES, 4 G PROTEIN, 8 G CARBOHYDRATE, 6 G TOTAL FAT (1 G SATURATED), 2 MG CHOLESTEROL, 150 MG SODIUM. EXCHANGE, EACH SERVING: 1/2 BREAD, 1 MEDIUM-FAT MEAT

Avocado Crisps

PREP TIME: 5 MINUTES   COOK TIME: 25 MINUTES

Chili Sauce

MAKES 2 CUPS (4 SERVINGS)

1 28-ounce can tomatoes

1 medium apple

1 medium onion

1 small green pepper

1 cup wine vinegar

1/2 cup sugar replacement

1 tablespoon salt

1/2 teaspoon ground clove

1/2 teaspoon cinnamon

1/2 teaspoon nutmeg

● Mash tomatoes; pour into kettle. Grind together apple, onion, green pepper, and vinegar. Add to kettle; cook until thick. Remove from heat. Add sugar replacement and seasonings. Return to heat; cook 5 minutes, stirring constantly.

EACH SERVING: ABOUT 106 CALORIES, 3 G PROTEIN, 27 G CARBOHYDRATE, 1 G TOTAL FAT (TRACE SATURATED), 0 MG CHOLESTEROL, 2,186 MG SODIUM. EXCHANGE, EACH SERVING: 1 FRUIT

PREP TIME: 10 MINUTES   COOK TIME: 6 MINUTES
(MARINATE OVERNIGHT)

Cheese-Bacon Crispies

MAKES 30 SERVINGS

1/4 cup low-calorie margarine, softened

1/4 pound Cheddar cheese, grated

1 teaspoon Worcestershire sauce

1/4 teaspoon Dijon mustard

2 tablespoons bacon bits

2/3 cup all-purpose flour

● Combine margarine, cheese, Worcestershire sauce, and mustard in a mixing bowl. Beat to blend. Add bacon bits and flour. Mix well. Form into a 1-inch-thick roll. Wrap in waxed paper and refrigerate overnight. Cut into 1/8-inch slices. Then bake on lightly oiled cookie sheet at 375°F for 6 minutes or until golden brown.

EACH SERVING: ABOUT 26 CALORIES, 1 G PROTEIN, 2 G CARBOHYDRATE, 1 G TOTAL FAT (TRACE SATURATED), 1 MG CHOLESTEROL, 60 MG SODIUM. EXCHANGE, 1 SERVING: 1/4 HIGH-FAT MEAT

PREP TIME: 10 MINUTES

Stuffed Celery

MAKES 1 SERVING

2 5-inch stalks celery

1 tablespoon cream cheese, softened

1/4 teaspoon onion powder

dash paprika

salt and pepper to taste

● Thoroughly rinse and drain celery. Combine cream cheese, onion powder, and paprika. Blend until smooth and creamy. Add salt and pepper. Fill celery stalks. Chill.

ABOUT 46 CALORIES, 2 G PROTEIN, 4 G CARBOHYDRATE, 3 G TOTAL FAT
(1 G SATURATED), 6 MG CHOLESTEROL, 80 MG SODIUM.
EXCHANGE: 1 FAT

PREP TIME: 10 MINUTES

Summer Chicken Canapés

MAKES 24 CANAPÉS (12 SERVINGS)

4 ounces chicken, ground and cooked

2 tablespoons margarine, softened

1/4 teaspoon dry mustard

1/4 teaspoon meat tenderizer

1/4 teaspoon salt

1/8 teaspoon pepper

1/8-inch-thick cucumber slices

● Combine chicken, margarine, dry mustard, meat tenderizer, salt, and pepper. Mix thoroughly. Chill. To make canapé: Place 1 teaspoon of chicken mixture in center of each cucumber slice.

PER SERVING: ABOUT 30 CALORIES, 2 G PROTEIN, 1 G CARBOHYDRATE,
2 G TOTAL FAT (TRACE SATURATED), 6 MG CHOLESTEROL, 80 MG SODIUM.
EXCHANGE, EACH SERVING: 1/2 FAT

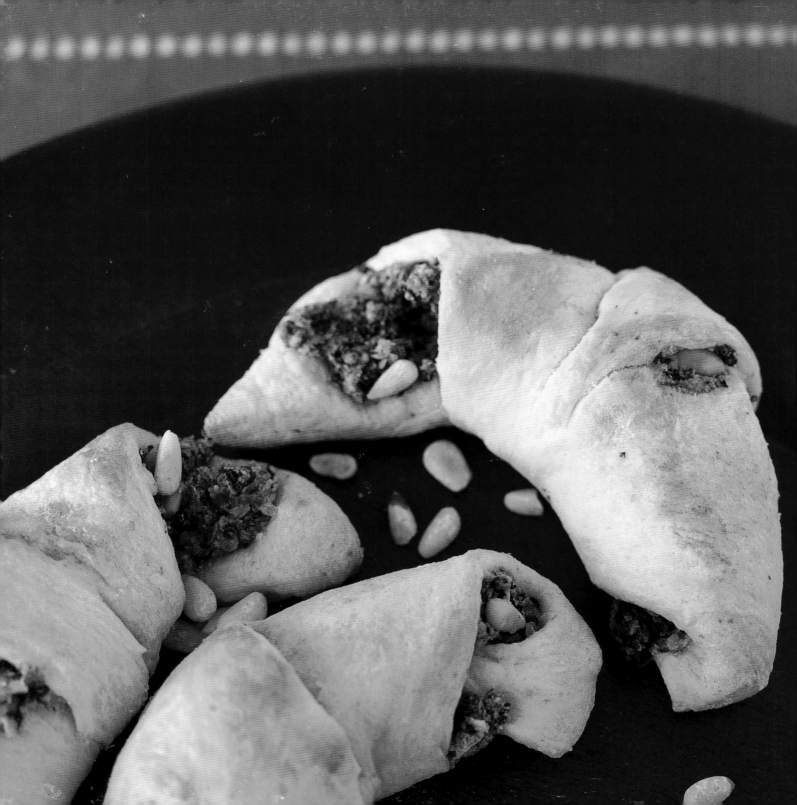

PREP TIME: 20 MINUTES   COOK TIME: 20 MINUTES

Spinach Crescents

MAKES 32 APPETIZERS

1/2 cup onion, finely chopped

2 tablespoons cooking oil

1 10-ounce package frozen chopped spinach,
thawed and squeezed dry

3/4 cup wheat germ

3/4 cup Parmesan cheese, grated

1/2 cup sour cream

1/4 cup pine nuts

1/2 teaspoon dried basil, crushed

1/4 teaspoon pepper

dash salt

2 8-ounce packages refrigerated crescent dinner rolls

1 egg white, beaten

● Sauté onion in hot oil for 2 to 3 minutes until tender. Remove from heat. Add the remaining ingredients except crescent rolls and egg white. Mix the filling thoroughly. Separate crescent rolls into triangles. Cut each triangle in half lengthwise. Spread 1 tablespoon of the filling, packed firmly, on each triangle. Roll up triangles, starting with the long end. Place on ungreased baking sheets. Brush with beaten egg white. Bake at 325°F for 16 to 18 minutes until golden brown. Serve warm.

EACH APPETIZER: ABOUT 83 CALORIES, 3 G PROTEIN, 10 G CARBOHYDRATE, 4 G TOTAL FAT (1 G SATURATED), 3 MG CHOLESTEROL, 120 MG SODIUM. EXCHANGE, EACH APPETIZER: 1/2 BREAD

PREP TIME: 10 MINUTES   COOK TIME: 3 MINUTES

Herbed Cheese on Toast

MAKES 24 SERVINGS

8 slices white bread

8 ounces cream cheese, softened

1 tablespoon skim milk

1 teaspoon onion, minced

1/4 teaspoon garlic, minced

1 teaspoon thyme

1 teaspoon sweet basil

1 teaspoon dill seed

salt and pepper to taste

● Toast the bread slices. Cut off crusts and cut each bread slice into three strips. Set aside. Combine remaining ingredients in a food processor or mixing bowl. Beat to blend thoroughly. Then spread mixture on toast fingers.

EACH SERVING: ABOUT 44 CALORIES, 2 G PROTEIN, 5 G CARBOHYDRATE, 2 G TOTAL FAT (1 G SATURATED), 6 MG CHOLESTEROL, 82 MG SODIUM. EXCHANGE, 1 SERVING: 1/4 STARCH/BREAD, 1/2 FAT

PREP TIME: 25 MINUTES   COOK TIME: 15 MINUTES
(MARINATE 24 HOURS)

Grilled Scallops

MAKES 24 SERVINGS

24 bay scallops

3 tablespoons olive oil

1/4 cup cider vinegar

2 cloves garlic, minced

2 teaspoons black pepper

2 large red bell peppers

12 slices bacon

● Combine scallops, oil, vinegar, garlic, and black pepper in a bowl. Cover and marinate for 24 hours. Peel and seed bell peppers, and then cut them into 2-inch squares. Place bell-pepper squares in a saucepan of boiling water. Reduce heat and allow to simmer for about a minute or until pepper is crispy-tender. Now cut bacon in half crosswise. Fry it over low heat until partially cooked but still limp. Place on a paper-lined plate to drain. Wrap one scallop and one red-pepper square in a bacon strip. Skewer with bamboo sticks or poultry pins. Grill until bacon is crisp.

PER SERVING: ABOUT 91 CALORIES, 3 G PROTEIN, 1 G CARBOHYDRATE, 8 G TOTAL FAT (3 G SATURATED), 11 MG CHOLESTEROL, 99 MG SODIUM. EXCHANGE, 1 SERVING: 1/2 MEDIUM-FAT MEAT

Grilled Scallops

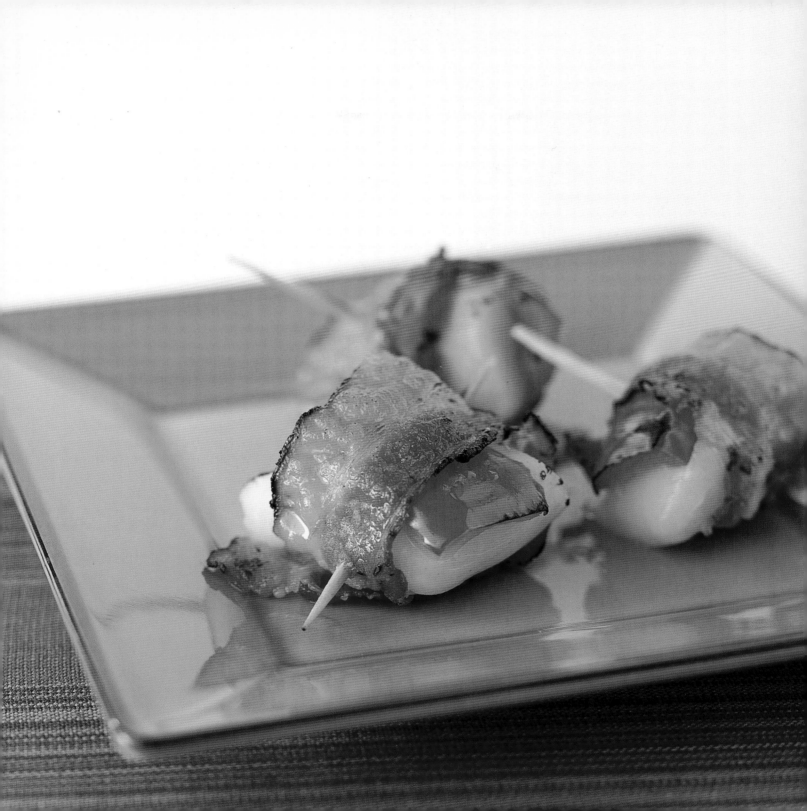

Potato-Crab Nibblers

MAKES 36 SERVINGS

1 cup prepared mashed potatoes

1 teaspoon dry minced onion

1 teaspoon Worcestershire sauce

1/8 teaspoon garlic powder

1 7 1/2-ounce can crabmeat, drained and flaked

1 egg, slightly beaten

1/2 cup dry bread crumbs

fat for deep-frying

● Combine prepared mashed potatoes, minced onion, Worcestershire sauce, garlic powder, and crabmeat in a bowl. Fold to completely blend. Shape into 36 bite-size balls. Dip into beaten egg; then roll in crumbs. Deep-fry in fat at 375°F for about a minute or until golden brown. Drain thoroughly.

EACH SERVING: ABOUT 33 CALORIES, 2 G PROTEIN, 2 G CARBOHYDRATE, 2 G TOTAL FAT (TRACE SATURATED), 11 MG CHOLESTEROL, 59 MG SODIUM. EXCHANGE, 1 SERVING: 1/4 STARCH/BREAD

Water Chestnut Nibbles

MAKES 16 SERVINGS

16 whole water chestnuts

1/4 cup soy sauce

4 slices bacon

● Drain water chestnuts thoroughly. Marinate in soy sauce for 30 to 40 minutes. Cut bacon in half both lengthwise and crosswise. Wrap a chestnut in each small slice of bacon. Secure with a toothpick. Arrange on a cookie sheet. Then bake at 400°F for 20 minutes. You can refrigerate to store, and reheat for 5 minutes before serving. This is a pop-in-the-mouth type of snack or appetizer.

EACH SERVING: ABOUT 44 CALORIES, 1 G PROTEIN, 3 G CARBOHYDRATE, 3 G TOTAL FAT (1 G SATURATED), 4 MG CHOLESTEROL, 299 MG SODIUM. EXCHANGE, 1 SERVING: 1/4 FAT

PREP TIME: 10 MINUTES

Onion-Cheese Ball

MAKES 40 SERVINGS

8 ounces cream cheese, softened
1 packet dry onion-soup mix

● Combine ingredients in a bowl. With an electric mixer, beat to thoroughly blend. Chill until you can work the mixture with your hands. Form it into a ball. Keep this in a bowl to nibble on.

**EACH SERVING: ABOUT 13 CALORIES, 1 G PROTEIN, 0 G CARBOHYDRATE,
1 G TOTAL FAT (1 G SATURATED), 3 MG CHOLESTEROL, 40 MG SODIUM.
EXCHANGE, 1 SERVING: 1/2 FAT**

PREP TIME: 30 MINUTES

Pastrami Roll-Ups

MAKES 12 SERVINGS

3-ounce package cream cheese, softened
2 tablespoons wine
1 tablespoon onion, minced
2 teaspoons horseradish
dash Worcestershire sauce
12 slices pressed pastrami

● Combine cream cheese, wine, onion, horseradish, and Worcestershire sauce in a bowl. Beat until blended and fluffy. Carefully unfold slices of pastrami, and flatten. Spread cheese mixture on pastrami slices. Then roll up as tight as possible. These freeze very well. Take them out of the freezer at least 15 minutes before serving time.

**EACH SERVING: ABOUT 58 CALORIES, 6 G PROTEIN, 1 G CARBOHYDRATE,
3 G TOTAL FAT (1 G SATURATED), 20 MG CHOLESTEROL, 329 MG SODIUM.
EXCHANGE, 1 SERVING: 1/2 MEDIUM-FAT MEAT**

Parsley Shrimp Ball

MAKES 40 SERVINGS

2 6-ounce packages frozen cooked shrimp

8 ounces cream cheese, softened

3 tablespoons finely chopped celery

1 clove garlic, minced

1 teaspoon soy sauce

1/4 teaspoon hot sauce

1/2 cup finely snipped fresh parsley

● Thaw, drain, and finely chop the shrimp. Combine shrimp, cream cheese, celery, garlic, soy sauce, and hot sauce in a bowl. Beat to blend. Chill until you can work it with your hands. Form mixture into a ball. Then roll it in finely snipped parsley.

EACH SERVING: ABOUT 22 CALORIES, 2 G PROTEIN, 0 G CARBOHYDRATE,
1 G TOTAL FAT (1 G SATURATED), 20 MG CHOLESTEROL, 53 MG SODIUM.
EXCHANGE, 1 SERVING: 1/3 MEDIUM-FAT MEAT

Asparagus Wraps

MAKES 10 SERVINGS

10 asparagus spears

2 tablespoons Dijon mustard

1 tablespoon reduced-calorie mayonnaise

10 slices proscuitto

● Trim the bottom end of the asparagus and blanch with boiling water. Blend the mustard and the mayonnaise in a small bowl. Divide and spread the mustard mixture evenly on the proscuitto slices. Wrap one asparagus spear in each proscuitto slice. Place the slices in a single layer on a round microwave platter or plate. Cover lightly with paper towels. With the microwave on Medium, cook for 1 minute or until hot; rotate the plate one-half turn after 30 seconds.

EACH SERVING: ABOUT 60 CALORIES, 6 G PROTEIN, 2 G CARBOHYDRATE,
4 G TOTAL FAT (1 G SATURATED), 17 MG CHOLESTEROL, 421 MG SODIUM.
EXCHANGE, 1 SERVING: 1 HIGH-FAT MEAT

Asparagas Wraps

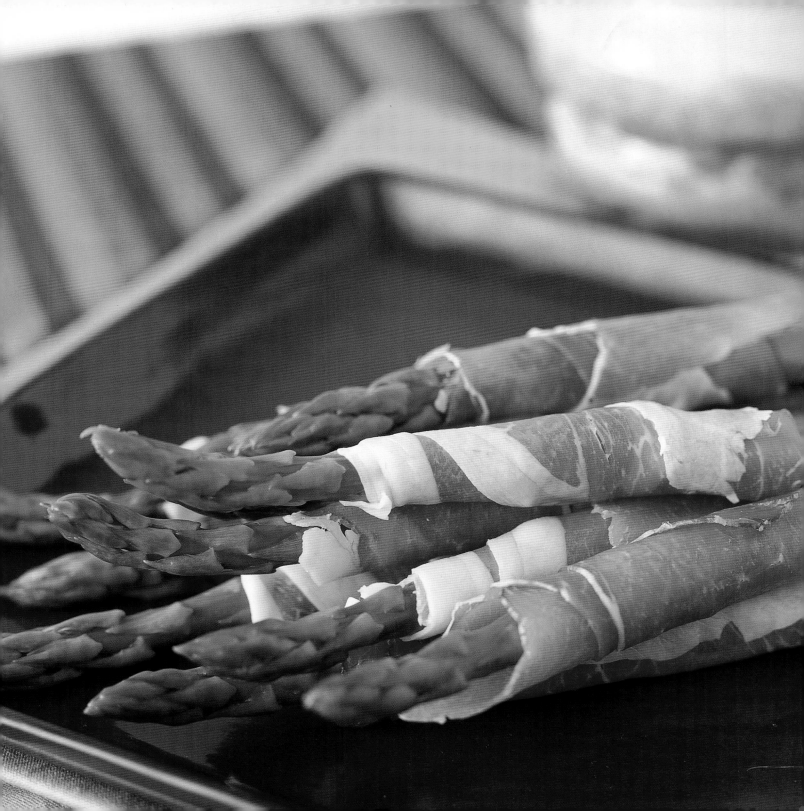

Shrimp Dip

MAKES 3/4 CUP

5 small shrimp, peeled, deveined, and cooked

1/2 teaspoon Worcestershire sauce

1 teaspoon lemon juice

4 ounces plain low-calorie yogurt

1/4 cup Chili Sauce (page 20)

● Crush shrimp. Sprinkle with Worcestershire sauce and lemon juice. Combine yogurt and Chili Sauce. Add crushed shrimp; stir to blend. Chill.

ABOUT 211 CALORIES, 15 G PROTEIN, 36 G CARBOHYDRATE, 3 G TOTAL FAT
(1 G SATURATED), 52 MG CHOLESTEROL, 2,480 MG SODIUM.
EXCHANGE: 1 MEAT, 1/2 MILK, 1/2 FRUIT

Smoked Salmon Canapés

MAKES 22 CANAPÉS (11 SERVINGS)

8 ounces smoked salmon

3 ounces cream cheese

1/2 teaspoon lemon juice

1 teaspoon milk

dash thyme

dash sage

salt and pepper to taste

● Place smoked salmon in blender. Blend until fine. Combine cream cheese, lemon juice, and milk. Stir to make a paste. Add seasonings. Mix well. Add salmon; blend thoroughly. Roll into 22 balls. Chill.

PER SERVING: ABOUT 42 CALORIES, 5 G PROTEIN, 0 G CARBOHYDRATE,
2 G TOTAL FAT (1 G SATURATED), 9 MG CHOLESTEROL, 194 MG SODIUM.
EXCHANGE, EACH SERVING: 1 MEAT

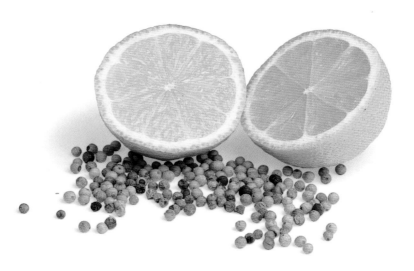

Hummus

MAKES 2 CUPS (8 SERVINGS)

1 1/2 cups chickpeas, cooked and drained,
  (liquid reserved)
1/2 cup tahini (ground sesame seeds)
1 clove garlic
3 tablespoons lemon juice
dash cayenne pepper
chopped parsley for garnish

● In the bowl of a blender, combine chickpeas, tahini, garlic, and lemon juice. Process until smooth. If mixture is too thick to blend well, add 1 tablespoon of reserved chickpea cooking liquid. Sprinkle cayenne over top, garnish with parsley, and serve with your favorite whole grain crackers.

EACH SERVING: ABOUT 138 CALORIES, 5 G PROTEIN, 13 G CARBOHYDRATE, 8 G TOTAL FAT (1 G SATURATED), 0 MG CHOLESTEROL, 14 MG SODIUM. EXCHANGE, EACH SERVING: 1 MEDIUM-FAT MEAT

Corn Relish

MAKES 3 CUPS (9 SERVINGS)

An old standby with lots of fiber.

1 cup vinegar
1/2 cup granulated sugar replacement
1 teaspoon dry mustard
1 teaspoon salt
1/4 teaspoon turmeric
2 cups canned whole kernel corn, drained
1/4 cup cabbage, finely chopped
1/2 cup onion, chopped
1/3 cup red bell pepper, chopped
1/4 cup green bell pepper, chopped

● Mix vinegar, sugar replacement, mustard, salt, and turmeric in a saucepan; heat to the boiling point. Add vegetables. Boil until vegetables are tender. Pour into serving dish and refrigerate until completely chilled.

EACH SERVING: ABOUT 49 CALORIES, 1 G PROTEIN, 12 G CARBOHYDRATE, TRACE TOTAL FAT (0 G SATURATED), 0 MG CHOLESTEROL, 385 MG SODIUM. EXCHANGE, EACH SERVING: 1/2 BREAD

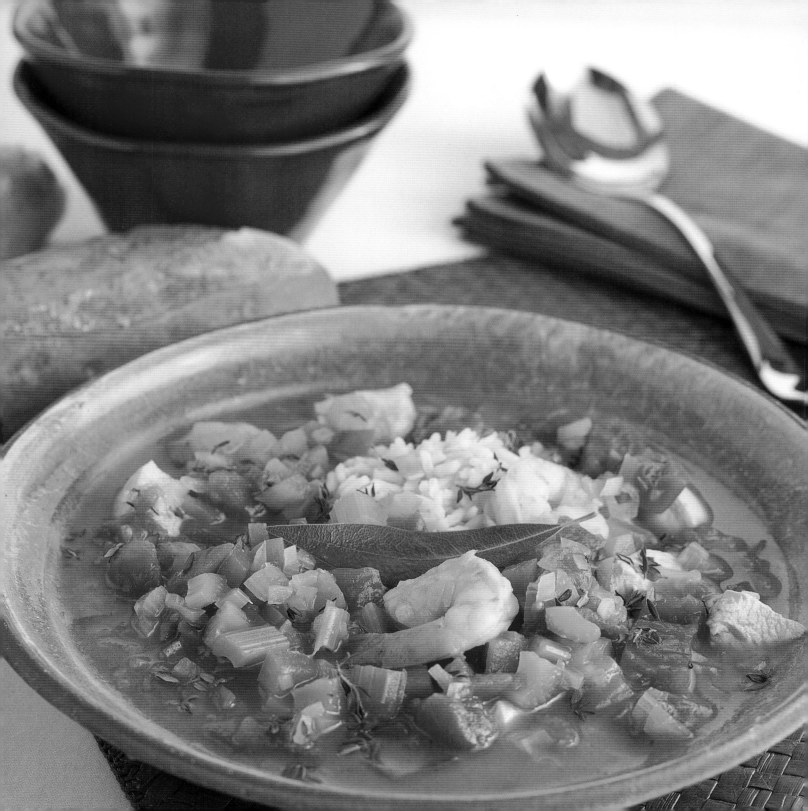

Soups & Stews

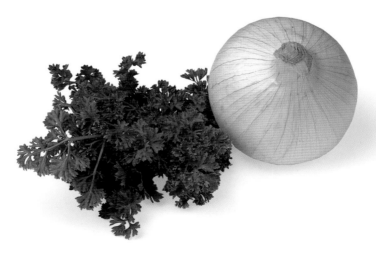

PREP TIME: 5 MINUTES   COOK TIME: 1 HOUR 30 MINUTES
(REFRIGERATE OVERNIGHT)

Chicken Broth

MAKES 2 QUARTS

2 pounds chicken, cut up

2 quarts cold water

1/2 medium stalk celery, chopped

8 to 10 green onions, chopped

2 tablespoons parsley, chopped

2 teaspoons salt

1 teaspoon thyme

1 teaspoon marjoram

1/2 teaspoon pepper

• Wash chicken pieces; place in large kettle. Cover with water; bring to boil, cover, and cook 1 hour or until chicken is tender. Add remaining ingredients; simmer 1 hour. Remove chicken; strain broth. Refrigerate broth overnight. Remove all fat from surface before reheating broth.

CALORIES: NEGLIGIBLE, EXCHANGE: NEGLIGIBLE

PREP TIME: 5 MINUTES   COOK TIME: 2 HOURS 30 MINUTES
(REFRIGERATE OVERNIGHT)

Beef Broth

MAKES 2 QUARTS

3 to 4 pounds beef soup bones or chuck roast

2 quarts cold water

1/2 stalk celery, chopped

3 carrots, sliced

1 medium onion, chopped

1/2 green pepper, chopped

2 bay leaves

1/2 teaspoon thyme

1/2 teaspoon marjoram

1/2 teaspoon paprika

1/2 teaspoon pepper

2 teaspoons salt

• Place beef in large kettle; cover with water. Bring to a boil, cover, and cook 2 hours, or until meat is tender. Add remaining ingredients; simmer 1 hour. Remove beef; strain broth. Refrigerate broth overnight. Remove all fat from surface before reheating broth.

CALORIES: NEGLIGIBLE, EXCHANGE: NEGLIGIBLE

German Cabbage Soup

MAKES 1¹/2 CUPS

2 ounces ground beef round

2 tablespoons onion, grated

dash mustard

dash soy sauce

salt and pepper to taste

1 tablespoon dry red wine

1¹/4 cups beef broth

2 large cabbage leaves, chopped

¹/2 medium tomato, cubed

¹/2 teaspoon fresh parsley, chopped

• Combine ground round, onion, mustard, soy sauce, salt, and pepper; mix thoroughly. Form into tiny meatballs. Add wine to broth; bring to boil. Add meatballs to broth, one at a time. Bring to boil again. Cook meatballs 5 minutes; remove to soup bowl. Add cabbage and tomato to broth. Simmer 5 minutes. Pour over meatballs. Garnish with parsley.

EACH SERVING: ABOUT 209 CALORIES, 15 G PROTEIN, 7 G CARBOHYDRATE, 13 G TOTAL FAT (5 G SATURATED), 43 MG CHOLESTEROL, 1,030 MG SODIUM. EXCHANGE: 1 MEDIUM-FAT MEAT, ¹/2 VEGETABLE

Cream of Chicken and Almond Soup

MAKES 1¹/2 CUPS

1 cup chicken broth

1 whole clove

1 sprig parsley

¹/2 bay leaf

pinch mace

1 tablespoon celery, sliced

1 tablespoon carrot, diced

1 teaspoon onion, diced

2 teaspoons stale bread crumbs

¹/2-ounce chicken breast

1 teaspoon blanched almonds, crushed

¹/4 cup skim milk

1 teaspoon flour

salt and pepper to taste

• Heat chicken broth, clove, parsley, bay leaf, and mace to a boil; remove from heat. Allow to rest 10 minutes; strain. Add celery, carrot, onion, bread crumbs, chicken, and almonds to seasoned chicken broth; simmer 20 minutes. In a small bowl, thoroughly combine skim milk and flour. Remove soup from heat; add milk mixture. Return to heat. Simmer (do not boil) 3 to 5 minutes. Add salt and pepper.

EACH SERVING: ABOUT 125 CALORIES, 12 G PROTEIN, 11 G CARBOHYDRATE, 4 G TOTAL FAT (1 G SATURATED) 10 MG CHOLESTEROL, 853 MG SODIUM. EXCHANGE: ¹/2 LEAN MEAT, 1 VEGETABLE, ¹/4 MILK

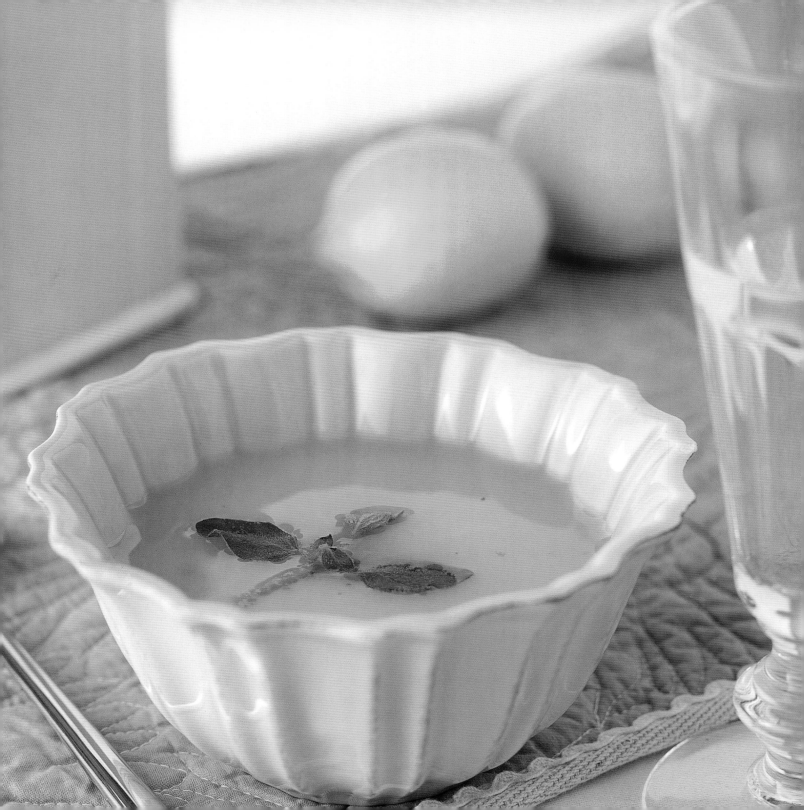

Greek Egg and Lemon Soup

MAKES 8 SERVINGS

2 quarts chicken broth

3 eggs, separated

juice of 1 lemon

● Bring broth to a boil in saucepan. Beat egg whites until stiff. Add egg yolks. Beat slowly until egg mixture is a light yellow. Add lemon juice gradually, beating constantly. Pour small amount of chicken broth into egg mixture. Then pour egg mixture into hot broth, beating constantly.

EACH SERVING: ABOUT 70 CALORIES, 7 G PROTEIN, 3 G CARBOHYDRATE, 3 G TOTAL FAT (1 G SATURATED), 80 MG CHOLESTEROL, 800 MG SODIUM. EXCHANGE, 1 SERVING: 1/4 HIGH-FAT MEAT

Ham and Split Pea Soup

MAKES 10 SERVINGS

2 pounds meaty ham bone

1 bay leaf

2 cups green split peas, dried

1 cup onions, chopped

1 cup celery, cubed

1 cup carrots, grated

salt and pepper to taste

● Cover ham bone and bay leaf with water. Simmer for 2 to 2 1/2 hours. Remove bone and strain liquid. Refrigerate overnight. Remove lean meat from bone; set aside. Remove fat from surface of liquid. Heat liquid; add enough water to make 2 1/2 quarts. Add peas; simmer for 20 minutes. Remove from heat and allow to stand 1 hour. Add onions, celery, carrots, and lean pieces of ham. Add salt and pepper. Simmer for 40 minutes. Stir occasionally.

EACH SERVING: ABOUT 369 CALORIES, 26 G PROTEIN, 27 G CARBOHYDRATE, 18 G TOTAL FAT (6 G SATURATED), 66 MG CHOLESTEROL, 63 MG SODIUM. EXCHANGE, 1 SERVING: 1/2 HIGH-FAT MEAT, 1 VEGETABLE

Greek Egg and Lemon Soup

French Meatball Soup

MAKES 1¹/2 CUPS

2 tablespoons rice

2 ounces ground beef round

1 tablespoon egg, beaten

1 teaspoon onion, grated

dash garlic

dash parsley

dash nutmeg

2 tablespoons dry red wine

1¹/4 cups beef broth

salt and pepper to taste

● Add rice to 1 cup salted water. Boil 5 minutes; drain well. Blend rice, ground round, egg, onion, garlic, parsley, and nutmeg; form into small meatballs. Add wine to broth; bring to a boil. Drop meatballs into hot broth, one at a time. Bring to boil again; reduce heat. Simmer 20 minutes. Add salt and pepper.

● Microwave: Add rice to 1 cup salted water. Bring to a boil. Hold 5 minutes; drain well. Combine meatball ingredients as above. Bring wine and broth to a boil. Drop meatballs into hot broth, one at a time. Bring to a boil again. Hold 10 minutes. Add salt and pepper.

EACH SERVING: ABOUT 242 CALORIES, 16 G PROTEIN, 7 G CARBOHYDRATE, 14 G TOTAL FAT (6 G SATURATED), 107 MG CHOLESTEROL, 1,038 MG SODIUM. EXCHANGE: 1 MEDIUM-FAT MEAT, 1/2 BREAD

Borscht

MAKES 4 SERVINGS

1 16-ounce can beets with juice

2 tablespoons sugar replacement

3/4 teaspoon salt

3 tablespoons lemon juice

1/2 teaspoon thyme

1 egg, well beaten

● Purée beets in blender. Add enough water to make 1 quart. Pour into saucepan. Add sugar replacement, salt, lemon juice, and thyme; heat to a boil. Remove from heat. Add small amount of hot beet mixture to egg. Stir egg mixture into beet mixture. Return to heat; cook and stir until hot. Added touch: top each serving with 1 teaspoon of low-calorie sour cream.

EACH SERVING: ABOUT 76 CALORIES, 3 G PROTEIN, 14 G CARBOHYDRATE, 1 G TOTAL FAT (TRACE SATURATED), 53 MG CHOLESTEROL, 669 MG SODIUM. EXCHANGE, 1 SERVING: 1 BREAD, 1/4 HIGH-FAT MEAT

Borscht

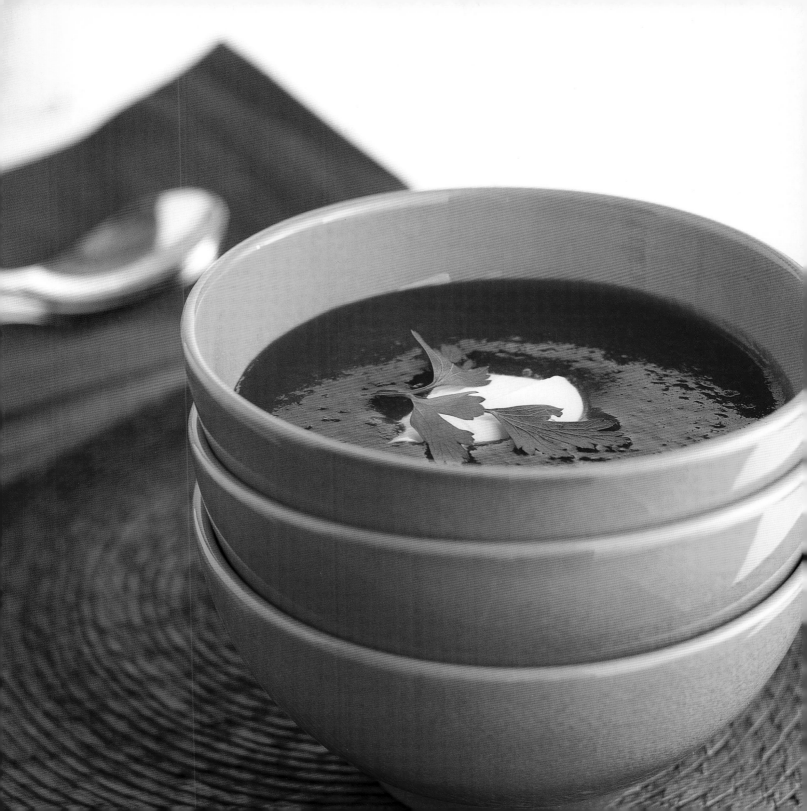

Crab Chowder

MAKES 1 CUP

1 cup milk

1 teaspoon flour

1/4 cup water

1/4 cup cooked crabmeat, flaked

3 tablespoons mushroom pieces

3 tablespoons asparagus pieces

salt and pepper to taste

● Blend milk, flour, and water thoroughly; pour into saucepan. Add crabmeat, mushrooms, and asparagus. Cook over low heat until slightly thickened. Add salt and pepper.

ABOUT 223 CALORIES, 26 G PROTEIN, 15 G CARBOHYDRATE, 6 G TOTAL FAT
(3 G SATURATED), 65 MG CHOLESTEROL, 1,034 MG SODIUM.
EXCHANGE: 1 MILK, 1 VEGETABLE, 1 LEAN MEAT

Oyster Soup

MAKES 1 1/2 CUPS

1 teaspoon flour

1 tablespoon celery, minced

1 teaspoon salt

dash Worcestershire sauce

dash soy sauce

1 tablespoon water

1 ounce oysters, with liquid

1 teaspoon butter

1 cup skim milk

● Blend flour, celery, salt, Worcestershire, soy sauce, and water in saucepan; add oysters with liquid, and butter. Simmer over low heat until edges of oysters curl. Remove from heat; add skim milk. Reheat over low heat.

EACH SERVING: ABOUT 164 CALORIES, 10 G PROTEIN, 16 G CARBOHYDRATE,
7 G TOTAL FAT (4 G SATURATED), 27 MG CHOLESTEROL, 2,530 MG SODIUM.
EXCHANGE: 1 LEAN MEAT, 1 MILK, 1/4 BREAD

**PREP TIME: 5 MINUTES   COOK TIME: 1 HOUR
(LET STAND OVERNIGHT)**

Bean Stew

MAKES 1 1/2 CUPS

1 tablespoon pinto beans

1 tablespoon great Northern beans

1 tablespoon lentils

1 cup beef broth

1 tablespoon carrot, sliced

1 tablespoon hominy

1 teaspoon diced onion

1/2 teaspoon green chilies, chopped

dash each garlic powder, oregano, salt, pepper

● Boil beans and lentils in beef broth for 10 minutes, covered. Allow to stand 1 to 2 hours, or overnight. Place softened beans and remaining ingredients in baking dish. Bake at 350°F for 45 minutes to 1 hour, or until ingredients are tender.

● Microwave: Place beans and lentils in beef broth; cover. Cook on High for 5 minutes. Allow to stand 1 to 2 hours or overnight. Add remaining ingredients. Cook on Medium for 10 to 15 minutes, or until ingredients are tender.

**ABOUT 95 CALORIES, 8 G PROTEIN, 14 G CARBOHYDRATE, 1 G TOTAL FAT
(TRACE SATURATED), 0 MG CHOLESTEROL, 883 MG SODIUM.
EXCHANGE: 1 LEAN MEAT, 2 BREAD**

PREP TIME: 10 MINUTES   COOK TIME: 1 HOUR

Pepper Pot

MAKES 1 SERVING

2 ounces lean pork, cut in 1-inch cubes

1 ounce beef, cut in 1-inch cubes

1 ounce chicken, cut in 1-inch cubes

1/4 cup carrot pieces

1/4 cup onion slices

1/4 cup celery pieces

1/4 cup potatoes, cubed

1/2 cup water

1 teaspoon flour

dash curry powder

dash garlic powder

salt and pepper to taste

● Brown pork and beef cubes slowly in frying pan. Add chicken cubes for last few minutes; drain. Place meat, carrots, onions, celery, and potatoes in an individual baking dish. Combine water, flour, and seasonings in screw-top jar; shake to blend well. Pour over meat mixture. Cover tightly and bake at 350°F for 45 minutes to 1 hour, or until meat is tender and gravy has thickened.

● Microwave: Reduce amount of water to 1/4 cup. Cover. Cook on High for 10 minutes. Hold 5 minutes.

**ABOUT 411 CALORIES, 34 G PROTEIN, 43 G CARBOHYDRATE, 11 G TOTAL FAT
(4 G SATURATED), 84 MG CHOLESTEROL, 117 MG SODIUM.
EXCHANGE: 4 HIGH-FAT MEAT, 1 VEGETABLE, 1 BREAD**

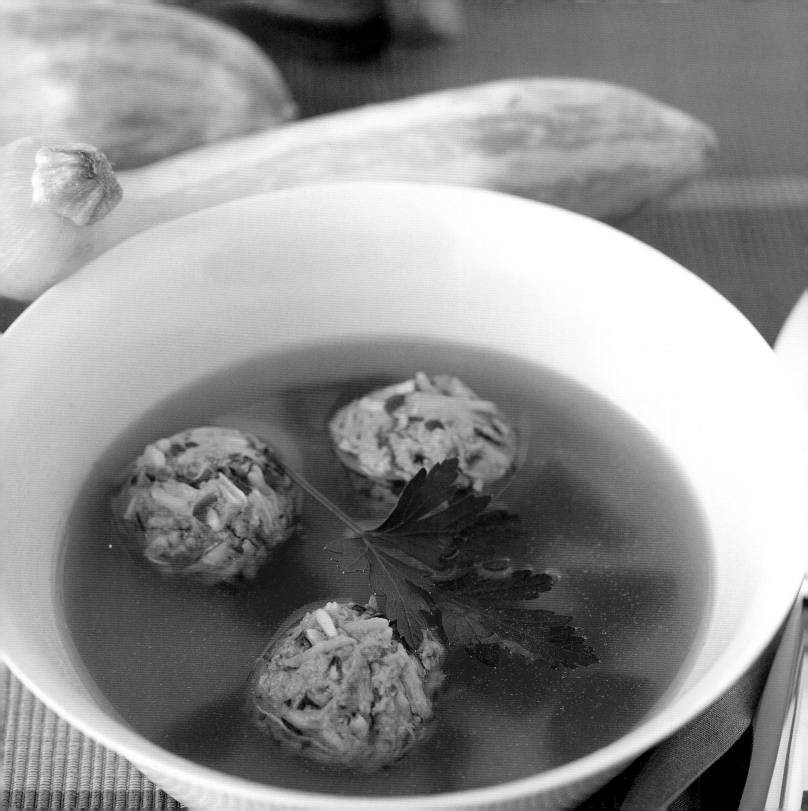

PREP TIME: 20 MINUTES   COOK TIME: 40 TO 50 MINUTES

Zucchini Meatball Stew

MAKES 1 3/4 CUPS

1 ounce ground beef

1/2 cup zucchini, ground

1 teaspoon onion, finely chopped

1 egg

1/4 cup rice, uncooked

dash oregano

dash cumin

dash garlic salt

dash pepper

1 cup beef broth

1 large tomato, diced

1 teaspoon parsley, chopped

salt and pepper to taste

● Combine ground beef, zucchini, onion, egg, rice, and seasonings; mix thoroughly. Shape into small meatballs. Combine beef broth, tomato, and parsley in saucepan; heat to boil. Drop meatballs into hot broth, one at a time. Cover and simmer 30 to 40 minutes. Add salt and pepper.

● Microwave: Cook beef broth, tomato, and parsley on High for 3 minutes, covered. Drop meatballs into broth. Cook on High 5 minutes. Hold 10 minutes. Add salt and pepper.

ABOUT 328 CALORIES, 23 G PROTEIN, 20 G CARBOHYDRATE, 17 G TOTAL FAT (6 G SATURATED), 446 MG CHOLESTEROL, 942 MG SODIUM. EXCHANGE: 2 MEDIUM-FAT MEAT, 1 VEGETABLE, 1 BREAD

Gazpacho

MAKES 4 SERVINGS

1/4 cup corn oil

1/2 cup onion, finely chopped

1 clove garlic, minced

11/4 cups tomato, peeled and chopped

1 cup green pepper, sliced into very thin strips

1/4 cup fresh parsley, chopped

dash hot pepper sauce

1/4 teaspoon dried basil

1/4 teaspoon oregano

dash black pepper

1 cucumber, halved lengthwise, seeded and very
   thinly sliced

1/2 cup chicken broth

1/2 cup water

1/3 cup dry white wine

● In a small saucepan, heat oil over medium heat. Add onion and garlic. Cook, stirring, for 2 minutes. In large bowl, stir together onion mixture and remaining ingredients. Combine all ingredients in a food processor fitted with a steel blade. Serve chilled.

EACH SERVING: ABOUT 177 CALORIES, 2 G PROTEIN, 9 G CARBOHYDRATE,
14 G TOTAL FAT (2 G SATURATED), 0 MG CHOLESTEROL, 108 MG SODIUM.
EXCHANGE, 1 SERVING: 2 VEGETABLE, 11/2 FAT

Cold Cucumber Soup

MAKES 4 SERVINGS

I happen to be a soup lover—so, a cold soup in summer is perfect.

2 large cucumbers

3 cups water

2 tablespoons cornstarch

4 chicken bouillon cubes

1 tablespoon white wine vinegar

1 tablespoon fresh dill, minced

1/2 cup low-fat plain yogurt

salt and pepper to taste

● Slice off ends of cucumbers; cut cucumbers into chunks. Combine 1 cup of the water and cucumber in blender or food processor. Mix together remaining water and cornstarch until blended. Combine cucumber and cornstarch mixture in a large soup pot. Add bouillon cubes, vinegar, and dill. Simmer and stir over low heat until bouillon cubes dissolve and mixture is hot. Remove from heat and cool slightly. Refrigerate, covered, until chilled. Stir in yogurt. Season with salt and pepper. Refrigerate until serving time.

EACH SERVING: ABOUT 58 CALORIES, 3 G PROTEIN, 9 G CARBOHYDRATE,
1 G TOTAL FAT (1 G SATURATED), 2 MG CHOLESTEROL, 767 MG SODIUM.
EXCHANGE, 1 SERVING: 1/3 NONFAT MILK

PREP TIME: 30 MINUTES   COOK TIME: 5 TO 6 HOURS
(LET STAND OVERNIGHT)

Russian-Jewish Barley Soup

MAKES 4 QUARTS

This recipe, given to me by my friend Sally Jordan, has been passed down through many generations of her family.

3/4 cup small lima beans

4 quarts water

1 1/2 pounds beef neck or chuck soup bone

1 cup celery, including leaves

1 onion, chopped

salt and pepper to taste

1 cup carrots, sliced

1 cup potatoes, diced

1/2 cup pearl barley

• Stovetop method: Place lima beans in mixing bowl; cover with 2 cups boiling water; soak overnight. In large soup pot, place soup bone, celery, onion, and enough water to completely cover the bone. Season with salt and pepper. Bring to a boil, reduce heat, and simmer until meat is very tender. Remove bone from soup pot and cut off all edible meat from the bone; return meat to the pot. Discard bone and membranes. Drain lima beans and add with the remaining ingredients to the soup pot. Adjust water to make 4 quarts of soup. Taste and season with salt and pepper. Cover and simmer for 5 to 6 hours.

• Slow-cooker method: Place lima beans in mixing bowl; cover with 2 cups boiling water; soak overnight. In a slow cooker, place soup bone, celery, onion, and enough water to completely cover bone. Add salt and pepper to taste. Cook on low during the night (8 to 12 hours). In the morning, remove meat from bone; discard bone and membranes. Drain lima beans and add with remaining ingredients to slow cooker. Add enough water to make 4 quarts of soup. Adjust salt and pepper to taste.

EACH 1 CUP SERVING: ABOUT 231 CALORIES, 10 G PROTEIN, 33 G CARBOHY-DRATE, 7 G TOTAL FAT (3 G SATURATED), 20 MG CHOLESTEROL, 42 MG SODIUM. EXCHANGE, 1 CUP: 1 BREAD, 1/2 MEDIUM-FAT MEAT

PREP TIME: 5 MINUTES   COOK TIME: 20 MINUTES

Chicken-Shrimp Gumbo

MAKES 8 SERVINGS

2 cups water

2 tablespoons instant chicken broth mix

1 16-ounce can whole tomatoes

1 cup celery, sliced

1/2 cup onion, chopped

2 bay leaves

1/2 teaspoon thyme

3 tablespoons all-purpose flour

1/2 cup sliced mushrooms (optional)

2 peppercorns (optional)

4-ounce boneless chicken breast

8 ounces uncooked shrimp, peeled and deveined

2 cups hot cooked rice

● Combine the water, chicken broth mix, and liquid from the tomatoes in a 3-quart casserole. Cook, uncovered, with the microwave on High for 2 minutes. Stir to dissolve the broth mix. Cut or chop the tomatoes. Add the tomatoes, celery, onion, bay leaves, and thyme to the liquid. Slowly stir in the flour. If desired, add the mushrooms and peppercorns. Cook, uncovered, with the microwave on High for 6 minutes. Reduce the heat to Medium Low, stir, and cook for 2 minutes longer. Remove the skin from the chicken breast, and cut the breast into large cubes or pieces. Add to the gumbo mixture. With the microwave on Medium, cook for 6 minutes. Cover and allow to rest for 5 minutes, or until the chicken is tender. Add the shrimp; then return soup to the microwave and cook on Medium for 4 minutes longer or until the shrimp is pink and thoroughly cooked. To serve: Place 1/4 cup of the hot cooked rice in the bottom of a large soup bowl. Ladle one-eighth of the gumbo on top.

EACH SERVING: ABOUT 134 CALORIES, 12 G PROTEIN, 18 G CARBOHYDRATE, 1 G TOTAL FAT (TRACE SATURATED), 51 MG CHOLESTEROL, 385 MG SODIUM. EXCHANGE, 1 SERVING: 2/3 BREAD, 1 LEAN MEAT, 1 VEGETABLE

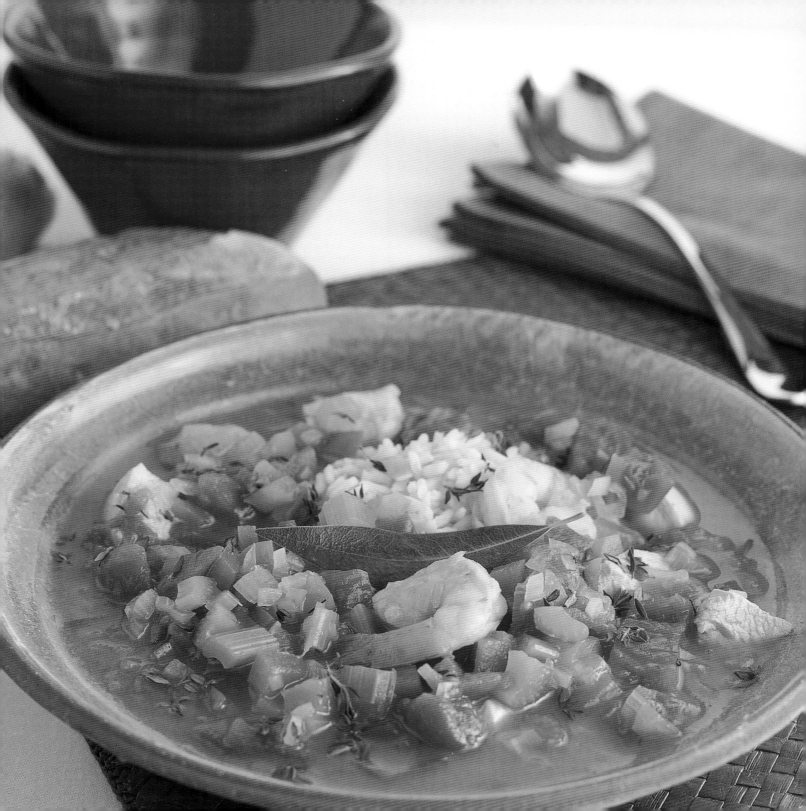

PREP TIME: 15 MINUTES   COOK TIME: 35 MINUTES

Tortilla Soup

MAKES 5 SERVINGS

Tortilla soup is a Mexican classic. Most tortilla soups contain cheese; some include meat. Tortilla chips take the place of bread croutons in this recipe. Aficionados who like the hot flavor of Mexican foods can add 1/2 teaspoon cayenne pepper to the blender ingredients.

3 tomatoes, peeled and halved

1 medium onion, coarsely chopped

1 clove garlic, minced

2 tablespoons fresh parsley or coriander (cilantro), chopped

1 15-ounce can tomato sauce

1/4 teaspoon honey

2 13 3/4-ounce cans chicken broth

2 teaspoons no-salt all-purpose seasoning

5 1/2 ounces baked tortilla chips

1 cup Cheddar cheese, grated

● In a blender, combine tomatoes, onion, garlic, parsley or coriander, tomato sauce, and honey. Cover and blend until nearly smooth. Pour into a large saucepan. Stir in the broth and seasoning; bring to a boil, cover, and simmer for 20 minutes. Divide tortilla chips among 5 soup bowls, sprinkle with cheese, and pour hot soup into the bowls over the cheese. Serve immediately.

EACH SERVING: ABOUT 263 CALORIES, 12 G PROTEIN, 32 G CARBOHYDRATE, 11 G TOTAL FAT (3 G SATURATED), 5 MG CHOLESTEROL, 1,143 MG SODIUM. EXCHANGE, 1 SERVING: 1 BREAD, 2 VEGETABLE, 1 HIGH-FAT MEAT, 1 FAT

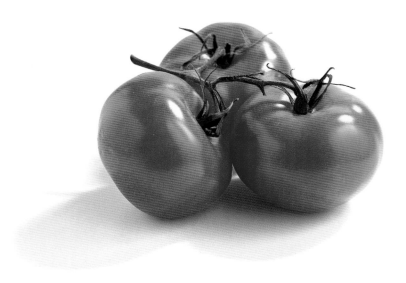

PREP TIME: 25 MINUTES   COOK TIME: 30 MINUTES

Asian-Inspired Minestrone

MAKES 6 SERVINGS

2 10³/4-ounce cans condensed chicken broth

1 soup can water

2 ounces spaghetti

1 clove garlic, minced

1 teaspoon gingerroot, grated

1 cup carrots, cut into julienne slices

1 cup broccoli stems, thinly sliced, and small florets

Wheat Germ Pork Balls (recipe follows)

1 cup fresh pea pods, halved

1 cup fresh spinach, romaine lettuce, or chard, chopped

● Heat together broth and water in a large saucepan until the boiling point. Stir in spaghetti, garlic, and ginger. Bring to a boil. Cover and simmer for 6 minutes. Add carrots and broccoli. Cover and simmer for 2 to 3 minutes until vegetables are crisp-tender. Add Wheat Germ Pork Balls, pea pods, and spinach, lettuce, or chard. Heat thoroughly.

● Microwave: Prepare Wheat Germ Pork Balls as directed above. Place in 1¹/2-quart glass baking dish. Microwave on high for 6 to 8 minutes or until meat is no longer pink, rotating once. Set aside. Place broth and water in a 3-quart glass casserole. Microwave on high for 9 to 10 minutes or until liquid boils. Stir in

spaghetti, garlic, and ginger. Microwave on high for 6 minutes. Add carrots and broccoli. Microwave on high for 2 to 3 minutes or until vegetables are crisp-tender and spaghetti is tender. Add Wheat Germ Pork Balls, pea pods, and spinach. Microwave on high for 1¹/2 to 2¹/2 minutes or until pea pods are crisp-tender.

EACH SERVING: ABOUT 213 CALORIES, 19 G PROTEIN, 23 G CARBOHYDRATE, 5 G TOTAL FAT (1 G SATURATED), 24 MG CHOLESTEROL, 788 MG SODIUM. EXCHANGE, 1 SERVING: 1 BREAD, 2 VEGETABLE, 1 HIGH-FAT MEAT

Wheat Germ Pork Balls

¹/2 pound lean ground pork

³/4 cup wheat germ

¹/2 cup water chestnuts, chopped

2 tablespoons soy sauce

2 tablespoons water

1¹/2 teaspoons gingerroot, grated

dash black pepper

● Combine all ingredients. Shape into 24 balls. Place in a large, shallow baking pan. Bake at 400°F for 20 minutes until lightly browned and thoroughly cooked. Cover and keep warm.

● Note: ¹/2 pound bulk pork sausage may be used instead of ground pork. Decrease soy sauce to 1 tablespoon and increase water to 3 tablespoons.

PREP TIME: 5 MINUTES   COOK TIME: 35 MINUTES

Krupnik

MAKES 8 SERVINGS

This is an American version of a very filling Polish soup. It is very tasty and quick to make.

1/2 cup pearl barley

2 quarts water

6 beef bouillon cubes

1 16-ounce package frozen mixed vegetables

1 2 1/2-ounce jar sliced mushrooms

3 medium potatoes, diced

1 tablespoon fresh parsley, chopped

2 teaspoons dillseed

2 egg yolks

● Cook barley as directed on package. Meanwhile, heat water and bouillon cubes in large soup kettle until cubes are dissolved. Add frozen vegetables, mushrooms, potatoes, 1 teaspoon of the parsley, and dillseed. Cook over medium heat until potatoes are tender. Add the cooked barley. Beat egg yolks with a small amount of water. A little at a time, stir egg yolks into soup mixture. Pour into a large soup tureen. Garnish with the remaining parsley.

EACH SERVING: ABOUT 177 CALORIES, 7 G PROTEIN, 33 G CARBOHYDRATE, 3 G TOTAL FAT (1 G SATURATED), 71 MG CHOLESTEROL, 655 MG SODIUM. EXCHANGE, 1 SERVING: 2 BREAD, 1/3 FAT

PREP TIME: 5 MINUTES   COOK TIME: 20 MINUTES

Vegetable Soup with Basil

MAKES 3 SERVINGS

1 cup water

2 teaspoons sweet basil

2 cloves garlic, sliced

1/2 bay leaf

1 10 3/4-ounce can vegetable soup

1 1/2 cups broken vermicelli noodles

● Combine water, basil, garlic, and bay leaf in a saucepan. Bring to a boil, reduce heat, and simmer for 5 minutes. Strain liquid. To the strained liquid, add vegetable soup and vermicelli noodles. While stirring, cook over low heat until noodles are tender.

EACH SERVING: ABOUT 104 CALORIES, 4 G PROTEIN, 20 G CARBOHYDRATE, 1 G TOTAL FAT (TRACE SATURATED), 0 MG CHOLESTEROL, 348 MG SODIUM. EXCHANGE, EACH SERVING: 1 STARCH/BREAD, 1/3 FAT

Savory Bean Stew

PREP TIME: 10 MINUTES   COOK TIME: 2 HOURS
(LET STAND 1 HOUR)

MAKES 5 SERVINGS

1 cup dry soybeans
1 quart water
1/3 cup onion, chopped
1 tablespoon margarine
1/2 pound ground beef
4 tomatoes, cored but not peeled
salt and pepper to taste

● Wash beans and combine with the water in a soup pot. Boil for 2 minutes. Cover and let stand for 1 hour. Simmer 1 to 1½ hours or until almost tender, adding water if necessary. In a casserole or pan, brown onion in margarine. Add beef, stir, and cook slowly for a few minutes. Cut tomatoes into small pieces. Add beans and tomatoes to the pot. Simmer until meat is tender and the flavors are blended, about 45 to 50 minutes. Season with salt and pepper.

EACH SERVING: ABOUT 240 CALORIES, 16 G PROTEIN, 11G CARBOHYDRATE, 16 G TOTAL FAT (5 G SATURATED), 34 MG CHOLESTEROL, 79 MG SODIUM. EXCHANGE, EACH SERVING: 1 BREAD, 1 1/2 MEDIUM-FAT MEAT, 1 VEGETABLE

Fresh Pea Soup

PREP TIME: 10 MINUTES   COOK TIME: 20 MINUTES

MAKES 10 CUPS

1 teaspoon vegetable oil
1 cup onion, chopped
1 cup carrots, shredded
4 cups iceberg lettuce, shredded
4 cups fresh peas, shelled
8 cups chicken broth
1 teaspoon salt
1/2 teaspoon black pepper

● In a large soup pot or Dutch oven, heat oil over medium heat. Stir in the onion and carrots. Cover and cook 5 minutes or until onion is translucent but not brown. Add remaining ingredients and bring to a boil. Cover, reduce heat, and simmer 10 to 15 minutes, stirring occasionally, until peas are tender. Remove from heat. Pour 2 cups of the soup into blender container. Cover and blend on low until mixture is puréed. Stir into the soup in the pot. Serve hot. (This soup freezes well for future use.)

EACH SERVING: ABOUT 96 CALORIES, 8 G PROTEIN, 12 G CARBOHYDRATE, 2 G TOTAL FAT (TRACE SATURATED), 0 MG CHOLESTEROL, 861 MG SODIUM. EXCHANGE, EACH SERVING: 3/4 BREAD

PREP TIME: 5 MINUTES   COOK TIME: 10 MINUTES

Fast, Fresh Cream of Tomato Soup

MAKES 6 SERVINGS

2 cups tomatoes, peeled and diced

2 tablespoons low-calorie margarine

2 tablespoons all-purpose flour

1 teaspoon salt

pepper to taste

1/4 teaspoon baking soda

1 cup skim milk

1/2 cup condensed chicken broth

● Combine tomatoes, margarine, flour, salt, and pepper in a blender. Blend on high until puréed. Pour into a saucepan. While stirring, cook until boiling. Reduce heat and simmer for 3 minutes. Stir in baking soda. Then gradually add milk and chicken broth. Heat thoroughly. Pour into six soup bowls.

EACH SERVING: ABOUT 88 CALORIES, 3 G PROTEIN, 10 G CARBOHYDRATE,
4 G TOTAL FAT (1 G SATURATED), 1 MG CHOLESTEROL, 829 MG SODIUM.
EXCHANGE, EACH SERVING: 1/3 LOW-FAT MILK, 1/3 VEGETABLE

PREP TIME: 5 MINUTES   COOK TIME: 15 MINUTES

Wild Rice and Mushroom Soup

MAKES 2 SERVINGS

1 cup condensed beef broth

1/2 cup thinly sliced mushrooms

1/2 cup cooked wild rice

1/3 cup water

2 tablespoons finely chopped onion

● Combine all ingredients in a saucepan. Bring to a boil, reduce heat, and simmer for 5 minutes or until mushrooms are tender.

EACH SERVING: ABOUT 73 CALORIES, 6 G PROTEIN, 10 G CARBOHYDRATE,
2 G TOTAL FAT (0 G SATURATED), 2 MG CHOLESTEROL, 1,147 MG SODIUM.
EXCHANGE, EACH SERVING: 1 STARCH/BREAD

Blanco Gazpacho

MAKES 4 CUPS

3 tomatoes, cut in chunks

1 large cucumber, peeled and cut into 2-inch chunks

3 tablespoons onion, chopped

1 slice whole wheat bread

2 cups water

1/2 cup chicken broth

2 tablespoons lemon juice

1 clove garlic

1 teaspoon salt

1/2 teaspoon black pepper

• Combine all ingredients in food processor fitted with a steel blade. Process on high speed, until mixture is smooth. Chill. Pour soup into bowls. Serve chilled. (This soup freezes well for future use.)

EACH SERVING: ABOUT 53 CALORIES, 3 G PROTEIN, 10 G CARBOHYDRATE, 1 G TOTAL FAT (TRACE SATURATED), 0 MG CHOLESTEROL, 721 MG SODIUM. EXCHANGE, EACH SERVING: 1 VEGETABLE

Green Bean Soup

MAKES 6 SERVINGS

3 cups green beans, cleaned and trimmed

3 cups chicken broth

1 cup carrots, cleaned and grated

3 green onions with tops, trimmed and chopped

1/2 teaspoon salt

1/3 cup low-fat plain yogurt

• Combine beans and 1 cup of broth in saucepan or Dutch oven. Bring to boil, reduce heat, and simmer until beans are tender. Remove from heat. Pour 1 cup of bean mixture into blender. Purée; return to pan. Add carrots, green onions, remaining broth, and salt to the soup. Simmer over low heat until mixture is hot. Remove from heat; stir in yogurt. Serve hot.

EACH SERVING: ABOUT 55 CALORIES, 5 G PROTEIN, 8 G CARBOHYDRATE, 1 G TOTAL FAT (TRACE SATURATED), 1 MG CHOLESTEROL, 601 MG SODIUM. EXCHANGE, EACH SERVING: 1 VEGETABLE

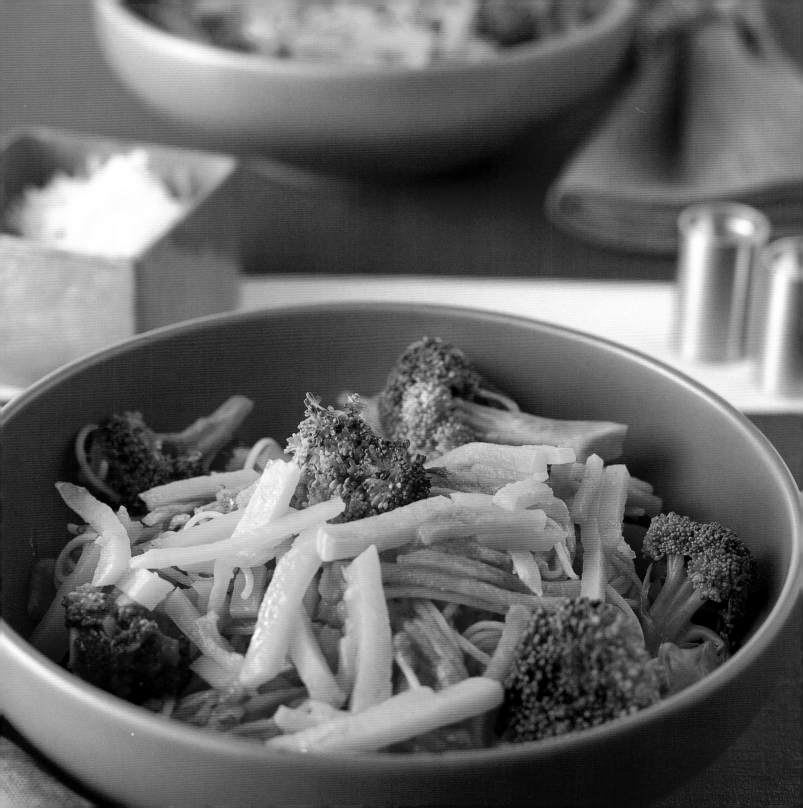

Pasta & Grains

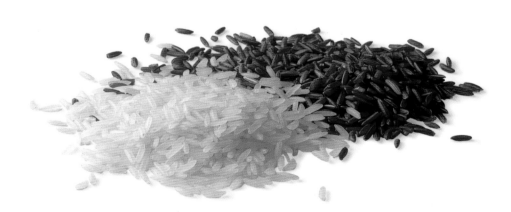

Clam Pilaf

MAKES 1 SERVING

2 ounces clams, minced
1/2 cup rice, cooked
2 tablespoons onion, chopped
1 medium fresh tomato, peeled and cubed
dash each ground bay leaf, thyme, salt, pepper
2 tablespoons grated Cheddar cheese

- Combine clams, rice, onion, tomato, and seasonings in baking dish; top with cheese. Bake at 350°F for 25 minutes.

- Microwave: Combine clams, rice, onion, tomato, and seasonings. Cook on High for 5 minutes; top with cheese. Reheat on High for 1 minute.

EACH SERVING: ABOUT 190 CALORIES, 12 G PROTEIN, 31 G CARBOHYDRATE, 2 G TOTAL FAT (1 G SATURATED), 21 MG CHOLESTEROL, 88 MG SODIUM. EXCHANGE: 2 LEAN MEAT, 1 BREAD

Crab Fried Rice

MAKES 6 SERVINGS

2 tablespoons margarine
2 eggs, lightly beaten
1 cup mushrooms, sliced
1 cup celery, sliced
1/2 cup onion, chopped
1/4 cup bamboo shoots
1/4 cup water chestnuts, sliced
3 cups brown rice, cooked
3 tablespoons soy sauce
1/2 pound crabmeat, cut in chunks

- Melt 1 tablespoon of the margarine in a large nonstick skillet. Add eggs and cook over low heat until set; remove to cutting board. Chop or cut eggs into large strips. Melt remaining 1 tablespoon margarine in the same pan. Add vegetables, cook, and stir until celery is tender. Remove vegetables from pan. Stir the rice into pan and add soy sauce. Mix until completely blended. Add vegetables, crab, and egg. Cover and cook over low heat until mixture is hot.

EACH SERVING: ABOUT 228 CALORIES, 13 G PROTEIN, 27 G CARBOHYDRATE, 7 G TOTAL FAT (1 G SATURATED), 87 MG CHOLESTEROL, 876 MG SODIUM. EXCHANGE, 1 SERVING: 1 BREAD, 1 VEGETABLE, 1 MEDIUM-FAT MEAT

Crab à la Lourna

MAKES 6 SERVINGS

This easy but elegant dinner was served the night our friend Lourna came to dinner.

2 tablespoons unsalted butter

1/2 pound small snow-white mushrooms

1/2 pound snow peas

1/2 pound crabmeat, cut into bite-size pieces

1 tablespoon all-purpose flour

1 teaspoon cornstarch

1 cup cold water

1/2 cup 2% milk

salt and pepper to taste

1 cup wild rice, cooked

2 cups brown rice, cooked

● Heat a large skillet and melt 1 tablespoon of the butter. Add mushrooms and sauté until tender; remove from heat. Meanwhile, clean snow peas and cut into 1-inch pieces. With a slotted spoon, remove mushrooms from skillet and return pan to medium heat. Add snow peas and cook until peas are tender; remove peas from pan. Melt remaining 1 tablespoon butter. Add crabmeat and sauté until lightly browned. Remove from pan. Dissolve flour and cornstarch in the water. Pour into skillet, add milk, and simmer over low heat until mixture thickens. Season with salt and pepper. Return the mushrooms, peas, and crabmeat to the pan. Heat and fold mixture gently until hot. Combine hot wild rice and brown rice. Serve Crab à la Lourna over the hot rice.

EACH SERVING: ABOUT 431 CALORIES, 19 G PROTEIN, 74 G CARBOHYDRATE, 7 G TOTAL FAT (3 G SATURATED), 28 MG CHOLESTEROL, 336 MG SODIUM. EXCHANGE, 1 SERVING: 1 BREAD, 1 VEGETABLE, 1 MEDIUM-FAT MEAT

PREP TIME: 15 MINUTES   COOK TIME: 30 MINUTES

Cheese Lasagna

MAKES 1 SERVING

1/2 cup Tomato Sauce (recipe follows)

3 tablespoons water

1 tablespoon minced onion

1/4 teaspoon garlic powder

1/2 teaspoon oregano

salt and pepper to taste

1/4 cup large curd cottage cheese

1 egg

11/2 cups lasagna noodles, cooked

2 ounces mozzarella cheese

1 tablespoon grated Parmesan cheese

● Combine Tomato Sauce, water, onion, garlic powder, oregano, salt, and pepper. Thoroughly blend together cottage cheese and egg. Spread small amount of sauce into bottom of individual baking dish. Alternate layers of noodles, sauce, cottage cheese mixture, and mozzarella cheese. Top with Parmesan cheese. Bake at 375°F for 30 minutes.

● Microwave: Cook on High for 10 minutes.

ABOUT 318 CALORIES, 18 G PROTEIN, 55 G CARBOHYDRATE, 3 G TOTAL FAT
(2 G SATURATED), 6 MG CHOLESTEROL, 609 MG SODIUM.
EXCHANGE: 3 HIGH-FAT MEAT

PREP TIME: 5 MINUTES   COOK TIME: 30 MINUTES

Tomato Sauce

YIELD VARIES

firm red tomatoes (or canned tomatoes without seasonings)

● Quarter the tomatoes. Place in large kettle. Push down with hands or back of spoon to render some juice. Bake at 325°F until soft pulp remains. Spoon into blender. Blend until smooth. Seal in sterilized jars or freeze.

PREP TIME: 5 MINUTES   COOK TIME: 5 MINUTES

Linguine with Clam Sauce

MAKES 12 SERVINGS

2 tablespoons olive oil

1 clove garlic, thinly sliced

1 tablespoon fresh parsley, chopped

1/2 teaspoon oregano

1 10-ounce can baby clams, with juice

8 ounces cooked linguine

• Combine the olive oil and garlic in a large measuring cup. With the microwave on High, cook, uncovered, for 3 minutes or until the garlic is slightly brown. Stir in the parsley, oregano, and clams with juice. Return to the microwave and cook on Medium for 2 minutes. Serve over the hot cooked linguine.

EACH SERVING: ABOUT 126 CALORIES, 9 G PROTEIN, 16 G CARBOHYDRATE, 3 G TOTAL FAT (TRACE SATURATED), 16 MG CHOLESTEROL, 28 MG SODIUM. EXCHANGE, 1 SERVING: 1 BREAD, 1/2 FAT

PREP TIME: 10 MINUTES   COOK TIME: 30 MINUTES

Fish Noodle Special

MAKES 1 SERVING

1/4 cup condensed cream of celery soup

2 tablespoons water

2 tablespoons mushroom pieces

2 tablespoons onion, finely chopped

dash thyme

dash ground rosemary

salt and pepper to taste

1 cup noodles, cooked

2 teaspoons peas

3 ounces cooked perch, flaked

• Blend condensed soup with water. Add mushrooms, onion, and seasonings; mix thoroughly. Combine noodles, peas, and perch in small baking dish. Pour soup mixture over entire surface; toss to mix. Bake at 350°F for 30 minutes.

• Microwave: Cook on High for 5 to 6 minutes.

EACH SERVING: ABOUT 335 CALORIES, 23 G PROTEIN, 47 G CARBOHYDRATE, 5 G TOTAL FAT (1 G SATURATED), 84 MG CHOLESTEROL, 530 MG SODIUM. EXCHANGE: 3 LEAN MEAT, 21/2 BREAD

PREP TIME: 5 MINUTES   COOK TIME: 30 MINUTES

Barley Hash

MAKES 4 SERVINGS

We like this for a quick lunch or supper. It is also a good recipe to help you use leftover beef.

1 1/2 cups water

3/4 cup quick-cooking barley

2 teaspoons salt

1/4 pound beef roast, cooked and cut into small pieces

1/4 cup onion, finely chopped

1/4 cup green pepper, finely chopped

2 tablespoons water

salt and pepper

● Bring water to a boil; stir in the barley and 2 teaspoons salt. Reduce heat, cover, and simmer for 10 to 12 minutes or until barley is tender; drain thoroughly. Meanwhile, combine beef, onion, and green pepper in nonstick skillet over medium heat. Add the water, cover, and heat until vegetables are tender. Drain off any excess water. Add barley and heat thoroughly. Season with salt and pepper to taste.

EACH SERVING: ABOUT 249 CALORIES, 11 G PROTEIN, 31 G CARBOHYDRATE, 9 G FAT (4 G SATURATED), 28 MG CHOLESTEROL, 1,175 MG SODIUM. EXCHANGE, 1 SERVING: 2 BREAD, 1 LEAN MEAT

PREP TIME: 5 MINUTES   COOK TIME: 30 MINUTES

Herbed Spinach Pasta

MAKES 5 SERVINGS

1/4 cup bran cereal

1/4 cup grated Parmesan cheese

dash black pepper

1/4 teaspoon dried basil

1/2 teaspoon oregano leaves

1 teaspoon fresh parsley, chopped

12 ounces spinach pasta ribbons

2 tablespoons margarine

● Crush cereal into crumbs. Stir in the cheese, pepper, basil, oregano and parsley. Set aside. Cook pasta ribbons according to package directions just until tender. Drain. Gently toss hot pasta with margarine. Add cereal mixture, tossing until well combined. Serve immediately.

EACH SERVING: ABOUT 227 CALORIES, 8 G PROTEIN, 32 G CARBOHYDRATE, 8 G TOTAL FAT (2 G SATURATED), 41 MG CHOLESTEROL, 107 MG SODIUM. EXCHANGE, 1 SERVING: 2 BREAD, 1/2 LEAN MEAT, 1 FAT

PREP TIME: 20 MINUTES   COOK TIME: 45 MINUTES TO 1 HOUR
(PLUS COOKING BEANS AND MILLET)

Soybean and Millet Casserole

MAKES 6 SERVINGS

1 cup soybeans

1 cup millet

1/2 cup onions, chopped

1/2 cup green pepper, chopped

3/4 cup mushrooms, chopped

1 teaspoon vegetable oil

2 eggs, beaten

2 tablespoons margarine

3/4 cup tomato juice

1 teaspoon fresh marjoram, chopped

1/4 cup brown sugar replacement

salt to taste

● Cook soybeans and millet according to package directions. Set aside. Sauté onions, green peppers, and mushrooms in the oil for 10 minutes. Mix in remaining ingredients. Bake in well-greased casserole at 325°F for about 45 to 60 minutes.

EACH SERVING: ABOUT 276 CALORIES, 12 G PROTEIN, 33 G CARBOHYDRATE,
11 G TOTAL FAT (2 G SATURATED), 71 MG CHOLESTEROL, 140 MG SODIUM.
EXCHANGE, 1 SERVING: 1 BREAD, 1 MEDIUM-FAT MEAT

PREP TIME: 5 MINUTES   COOK TIME: 25 TO 30 MINUTES

Golden Barley

MAKES 4 SERVINGS

You don't always have to serve potatoes. Try barley for a new side dish.

1/2 cup Cheddar cheese soup

2 tablespoons hot water

1 tablespoon ketchup

1 1/2 cups cooked barley

1/4 cup fresh parsley, chopped

● Combine cheese soup, hot water, and ketchup in a mixing bowl. Stir to blend. Add barley and thoroughly mix. Spoon into a greased microwave baking dish. Cover tightly. Microwave on Medium for 7 minutes. Turn dish and stir slightly. Return to microwave; cook 3 minutes more. Remove cover, and garnish with parsley.

● Oven method: Increase water to 1/4 cup. Combine as above. Spoon into a greased baking dish or casserole. Cover tightly. Bake at 350°F for 25 to 30 minutes or until mixture is bubbly. Garnish with parsley.

EACH SERVING: ABOUT 103 CALORIES, 3 G PROTEIN, 19 G CARBOHYDRATE,
2 G TOTAL FAT (1 G SATURATED), 6 MG CHOLESTEROL, 131 MG SODIUM.
EXCHANGE, 1 SERVING: 1 BREAD

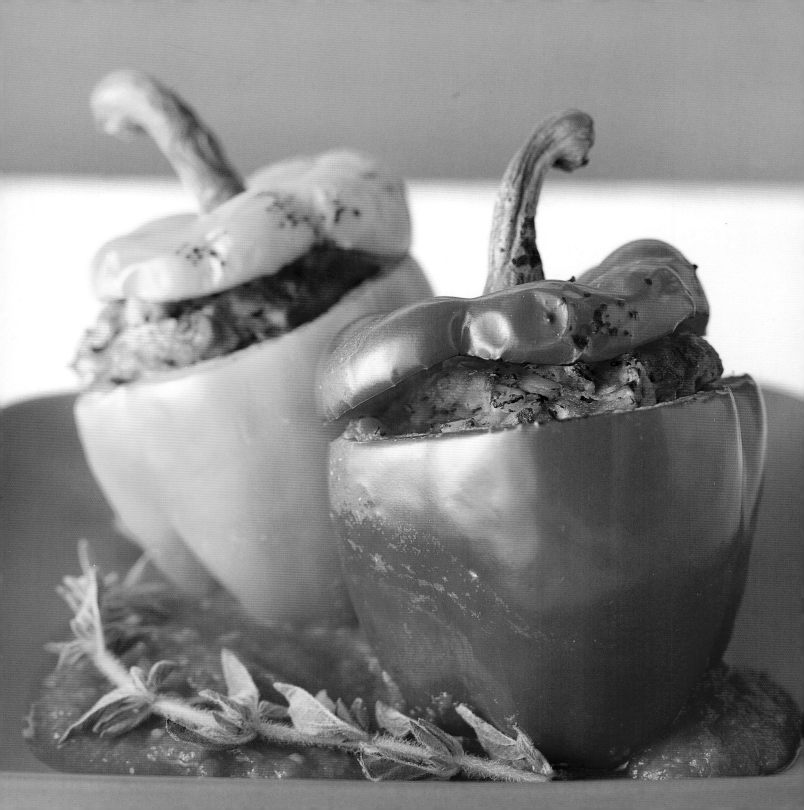

Stuffed Pepper

MAKES 1 SERVING

1 green, red, or yellow bell pepper

2 tablespoons rice

1/2 cup water

2 ounces lean ground beef

1 egg

1 teaspoon onion flakes

1 tablespoon mushrooms, finely chopped

salt and pepper to taste

1 teaspoon Tomato Sauce (page 58)

● Cut top off bell pepper; reserve. Remove membrane and seeds; rinse, drain, and reserve shells. Boil rice with 1/2 cup of water for 5 minutes; drain. Combine ground beef, rice, egg, onion flakes, and mushrooms; blend thoroughly. Add salt and pepper. Fill bell pepper cavity with beef mixture; top with Tomato Sauce. Top stuffed pepper with reserved bell pepper top. Place in baking dish; cover. Bake at 350°F for 20 to 25 minutes.

● Microwave: Cook on High for 10 minutes.

EACH SERVING: ABOUT 289 CALORIES, 18 G PROTEIN, 15 G CARBOHYDRATE, 17 G TOTAL FAT (6 G SATURATED), 255 MG CHOLESTEROL, 140 MG SODIUM. EXCHANGE: 3 MEDIUM-FAT MEAT, 1 BREAD, 1 VEGETABLE

Baked Rice

MAKES 1 SERVING

1 cube beef bouillon

1 cup hot water

1/4 cup rice

1 green onion, chopped

2 tablespoons celery, chopped

3 tablespoons dry bread crumbs

● Dissolve bouillon in hot water. Add rice, green onion, and celery; cover. Cook for 5 minutes. Add bread crumbs. Pour into small baking dish. Bake at 350°F for 25 to 30 minutes, or until top is lightly crusted.

EACH SERVING: ABOUT 147 CALORIES, 5 G PROTEIN, 28 G CARBOHYDRATE, 2 G TOTAL FAT (TRACE SATURATED), 0 MG CHOLESTEROL, 802 MG SODIUM. EXCHANGE: 1 1/2 BREAD

Stuffed Pepper

PREP TIME: 20 MINUTES   COOK TIME: 30 MINUTES

Veal Scaloppine I

MAKES 1 SERVING

1/2 teaspoon margarine

2 ounces veal round steak, thinly sliced

2 tablespoons tomato paste

6 tablespoons water

salt and pepper to taste

dash oregano

dash garlic powder

1 tablespoon mushrooms, sliced

1 teaspoon onion, chopped

1 cup cooked spaghetti

• Melt margarine in small skillet. Brown both sides of veal steaks slices. Place in small baking dish. Blend tomato paste, water, seasonings, mushrooms, and onion together. Pour over veal; cover. Bake at 350°F for 30 minutes. Place veal on top of spaghetti. Pour sauce over all.

• Microwave: Cook covered on Medium for 12 minutes.

ABOUT 377 CALORIES, 25 G PROTEIN, 47 G CARBOHYDRATE, 10 G TOTAL FAT
(3 G SATURATED), 15 MG CHOLESTEROL, 310 MG SODIUM.
EXCHANGE: 2 MEDIUM-FAT MEAT, 2 BREAD

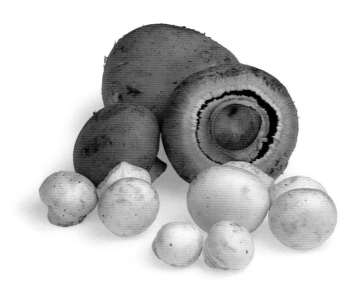

PREP TIME: 30 MINUTES   COOK TIME: 40 MINUTES

Macaroni and Cheese Supreme

MAKES 6 SERVINGS

1 cup elbow macaroni

1 11-ounce can condensed cream of mushroom soup

6 ounces cheese, shredded

1 teaspoon yellow mustard

1 teaspoon salt

dash pepper

2 cups cooked spinach, drained

12 ounces lean meat, diced

● Cook macaroni as directed on package; drain. Combine mushroom soup, cheese, mustard, salt, and pepper. Add macaroni; stir well. Spread cooked spinach on bottom of lightly greased 13" x 9" baking dish. Top with meat. Spoon macaroni mixture evenly over entire surface. Bake at 375°F for 40 minutes. Allow to cool 15 minutes before serving.

● Microwave: Cook on Medium for 12 to 15 minutes. Turn dish halfway through cooking time. Allow to rest 15 minutes before serving.

EACH SERVING: ABOUT 219 CALORIES, 23 G PROTEIN, 15 G CARBOHYDRATE, 7 G TOTAL FAT (3 G SATURATED), 39 MG CHOLESTEROL, 581 MG SODIUM. EXCHANGE, 1 SERVING: 2 BREAD, 3 HIGH-FAT MEAT, 1 VEGETABLE

PREP TIME: 10 MINUTES   COOK TIME: 20 MINUTES

Great Spaghetti

MAKES 4 SERVINGS

2 tomatoes

1/4 cup garlic chives, chopped

1/4 cup green pepper, chopped

water

2 cups cooked spaghetti noodles

salt and pepper to taste

● Core the unpeeled tomatoes; chop or cut into small pieces. Place in a medium saucepan. Add chives, green pepper, and a small amount of water. Cover and cook until tomatoes are tender. Add cooked spaghetti. Stir to completely coat spaghetti. Simmer over low heat until spaghetti is hot. Season with salt and pepper.

EACH SERVING: ABOUT 146 CALORIES, 2 G PROTEIN, 24 G CARBOHYDRATE, 5 G TOTAL FAT (1 G SATURATED), 0 MG CHOLESTEROL, 1,156 MG SODIUM. EXCHANGE, 1 SERVING: 1 BREAD, 1 VEGETABLE

Rice Pilaf

MAKES 1 CUP

1/2 cup rice

1 teaspoon butter

1/2 teaspoon salt

1 tablespoon lemon juice

1 cup boiling water

• Sauté rice in butter over low heat in large saucepan. Add remaining ingredients. Bring to a boil. Reduce heat; cover. Simmer until water is absorbed. Fluff with fork before serving.

ABOUT 146 CALORIES, 2 G PROTEIN, 24 G CARBOHYDRATE, 5 G TOTAL FAT (1 G SATURATED), 0 MG CHOLESTEROL, 1,156 MG SODIUM. EXCHANGE: 2 BREAD, 1 FAT

Wild Rice

MAKES 14 SERVINGS

1 pound long-grain wild rice

1 quart water

salt

1/2 cup dried cranberries, optional

1/2 cup walnuts, optional

• Combine the rice, water, and salt in a 3-quart casserole with a cover. With the microwave on High, cook for 5 minutes. Stir to mix. Still on High, cook for 5 minutes; then rotate the casserole one-quarter turn. Cook on High for 5 more minutes. The rice should show the white kernel on the inside. If desired, mix in the dried cranberries and walnuts. Allow to set for 10 to 15 minutes.

• To package for the freezer: Drain the rice in a strainer and cool it with running water. Allow to drain. Spoon 1 cup of the cooled rice into small freezer bags for future use.

EACH SERVING: ABOUT 116 CALORIES, 5 G PROTEIN, 24 G CARBOHYDRATE, TRACE TOTAL FAT (TRACE SATURATED), 0 MG CHOLESTEROL, 2 MG SODIUM. EXCHANGE, 1/3 CUP: 1 BREAD

Wild Rice

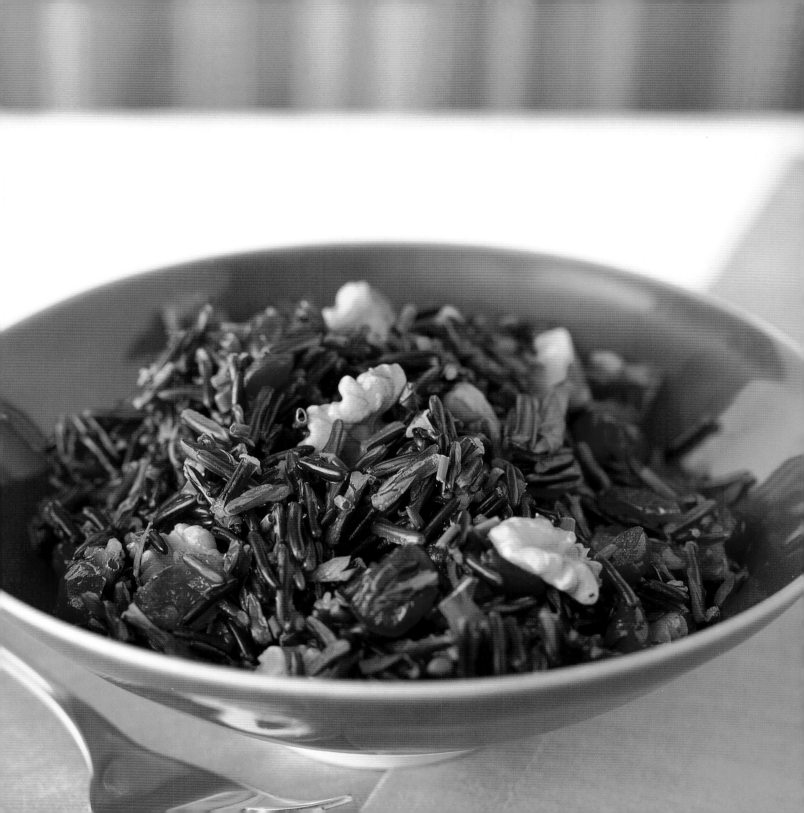

PREP TIME: 20 MINUTES   COOK TIME: 15 MINUTES

Savory Bran-Rice Pilaf

MAKES 6 SERVINGS

1/2 cup long-grain brown rice

1 chicken bouillon cube

1/4 cup margarine

1/4 cup onion, chopped

1/2 cup celery, chopped

1/2 cup mushrooms, sliced and drained

1/4 cup water chestnuts, sliced

1 cup bran cereal

1/4 teaspoon ground sage

1/2 teaspoon dried basil

dash pepper

1/2 cup water

● Cook rice according to package directions, adding the bouillon cube instead of the salt and butter called for in the directions. While rice is cooking, melt margarine in a large skillet. Stir in onion, celery, mushrooms, and water chestnuts. Cook over medium heat, stirring occasionally, until celery is almost tender. Gently stir in the cooked rice, cereal, sage, basil, pepper, and water. Cover and cook over very low heat about 15 minutes. Serve immediately.

EACH SERVING: ABOUT 183 CALORIES, 3 G PROTEIN, 24 G CARBOHYDRATE, 10 G TOTAL FAT (1 G SATURATED), 0 MG CHOLESTEROL, 176 MG SODIUM. EXCHANGE, 1 SERVING: 1 BREAD, 1 VEGETABLE, 2 FAT

PREP TIME: 10 MINUTES   COOK TIME: 15 MINUTES

Bulgur Pilaf

MAKES 4 SERVINGS

1 tablespoon margarine

1 cup bulgur wheat

2 cups beef broth, hot

1/4 cup chives, chopped

3 tablespoons sweet red pepper

3 tablespoons fresh parsley, chopped

salt and pepper to taste

● Melt margarine in a medium saucepan. Add bulgur and sauté for 1 minute, stirring constantly. Add broth, chives, and red pepper. Stir to mix. Simmer, covered, over low heat for 15 minutes or until broth is absorbed. Stir in parsley. Season with salt and pepper. Spoon into serving dish.

EACH SERVING: ABOUT 162 CALORIES, 6 G PROTEIN, 27 G CARBOHYDRATE, 4 G TOTAL FAT (1 G SATURATED), 0 MG CHOLESTEROL, 399 MG SODIUM. EXCHANGE, 1 SERVING: 2 BREAD

PREP TIME: 10 MINUTES   COOK TIME: 20 MINUTES

Broccoli & Pasta with Cheese

MAKES 8 SERVINGS

1¹/4 pounds fresh broccoli

2 tablespoons salt

8 ounces small shell pasta

16 cherry tomatoes, halved

1 clove garlic, minced

¹/4 cup Parmesan cheese, grated

• Cut florets from broccoli head and slice stems crosswise into ¹/2-inch pieces. In a large saucepan, heat 2 quarts water to the boiling point. Add broccoli and 1 tablespoon of the salt. Cook 4 to 5 minutes or until crisp-tender. Drain in strainer or colander. In the same pan, bring 3 quarts water to the boiling point. Add pasta and 1 tablespoon salt to water; cook until pasta is al dente ("firm to the teeth"). Remove from heat but do not drain. Add tomato halves and garlic to hot pasta and water. Cover and allow to rest for 5 minutes. Add broccoli and reheat slightly. Drain in strainer or colander. While in strainer, sprinkle mixture with half the cheese, toss lightly, and repeat with remaining cheese. Pour into hot serving bowl.

EACH SERVING: ABOUT 144 CALORIES, 7 G PROTEIN, 27 G CARBOHYDRATE, 2 G TOTAL FAT (1 G SATURATED), 2 MG CHOLESTEROL, 1,815 MG SODIUM. EXCHANGE, 1 SERVING: 1 BREAD, 1 VEGETABLE, 1 FAT

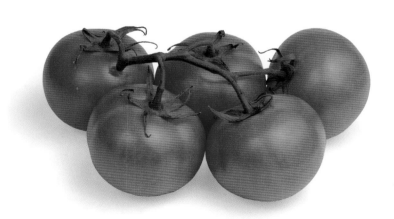

PREP TIME: 5 MINUTES   COOK TIME: 15 MINUTES

Mostaccioli with Oysters

MAKES 2 SERVINGS

1 8-ounce can oysters with liquid, minced

1 4-ounce can mushroom pieces

1/2 cup green pepper, sliced

1 tablespoon parsley

1 teaspoon garlic powder

salt and pepper to taste

3 cups mostaccioli noodles, cooked

• Combine minced oysters with liquid, mushrooms, green pepper, and parsley in saucepan. Add garlic powder. Cook until green pepper is crispy but tender. Add salt and pepper. Serve over mostaccioli noodles.

• Microwave: Combine minced oysters with liquid, mushrooms, green pepper, parsley, and garlic powder in bowl. Cook on High for 4 minutes or until green pepper is crispy but tender. Add salt and pepper. Serve over mostaccioli noodles.

EACH SERVING: ABOUT 411 CALORIES, 21 G PROTEIN, 71 G CARBOHYDRATE, 5 G TOTAL FAT (1 G SATURATED), 68 MG CHOLESTEROL, 384 MG SODIUM. EXCHANGE, 1 SERVING: 4 LEAN MEAT, 1 1/2 BREAD

PREP TIME: 5 MINUTES   COOK TIME: 20 MINUTES

Vegetable Angel Hair Pasta

MAKES 6 SERVINGS

1 12-ounce package angel hair pasta

4 small stalks broccoli, thinly sliced lengthwise

1 medium butternut squash, peeled and thinly sliced

1 large carrot, shredded

1 tablespoon onion, chopped

1 32-ounce jar meatless spaghetti sauce

1/2 cup Parmesan cheese, grated

1/2 cup bean sprouts

• Cook angel hair as package directs for 7 minutes. Add vegetables; cook 5 minutes and drain. In a medium saucepan, simmer spaghetti sauce for 5 minutes or until thoroughly heated. Place pasta and vegetables in a large bowl. Add sauce and cheese; toss well. Serve 6 equal portions topped with the bean sprouts.

EACH SERVING: ABOUT 313 CALORIES, 13 G PROTEIN, 60 G CARBOHYDRATE, 3 G TOTAL FAT (1 G SATURATED), 5 MG CHOLESTEROL, 1,051 MG SODIUM. EXCHANGE, 1 SERVING: 3 1/2 BREAD, 2 VEGETABLE, 1 MEDIUM-FAT MEAT

Vegetable Angel Hair Pasta

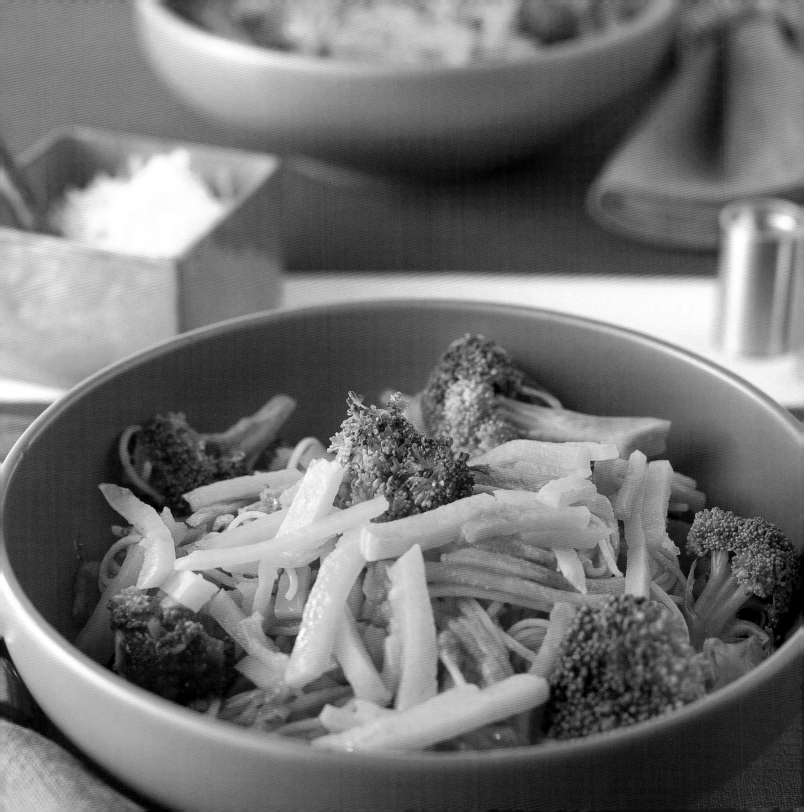

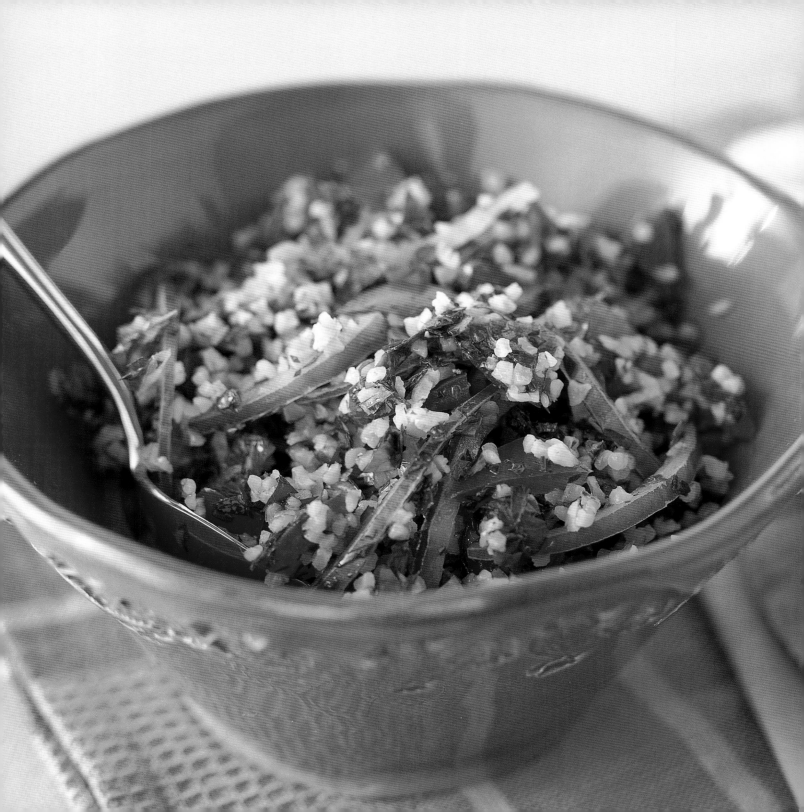

Tabbouleh

MAKES 8 SERVINGS

1/2 cup cracked wheat

3 medium fresh tomatoes, finely chopped

1 cup parsley, finely chopped

1 red onion, sliced

1/3 cup fresh lemon juice

2 teaspoons salt

1 tablespoon vegetable oil

● Soak cracked wheat in cold water for about 10 minutes; drain. Wrap in cheese cloth and squeeze until dry. In large bowl, combine cracked wheat, tomatoes, parsley, onion, lemon juice, and salt; toss lightly with a fork. Marinate at least half an hour before serving. Just before serving, stir in the oil.

EACH SERVING: ABOUT 67 CALORIES, 2 G PROTEIN, 12 G CARBOHYDRATE, 2 G TOTAL FAT (TRACE SATURATED), 0 MG CHOLESTEROL, 588 MG SODIUM. EXCHANGE, 1 SERVING: 2/3 BREAD, 1/2 FAT

Cheese & Rice Balls

MAKES 8 SERVINGS

1 cup cooked rice

1/4 cup grated Romano cheese

1/4 cup grated Parmesan cheese

1 egg, beaten

1 teaspoon horseradish

● Combine all ingredients; then stir to blend thoroughly. Form into eight balls. In a skillet sprayed with vegetable oil, sauté until lightly browned.

EACH SERVING: ABOUT 58 CALORIES, 3 G PROTEIN, 6 G CARBOHYDRATE, 2 G TOTAL FAT (1 G SATURATED), 31 MG CHOLESTEROL, 103 MG SODIUM. EXCHANGE, EACH SERVING: 1/2 MEDIUM-FAT MEAT, 1/4 STARCH/BREAD

Tabbouleh

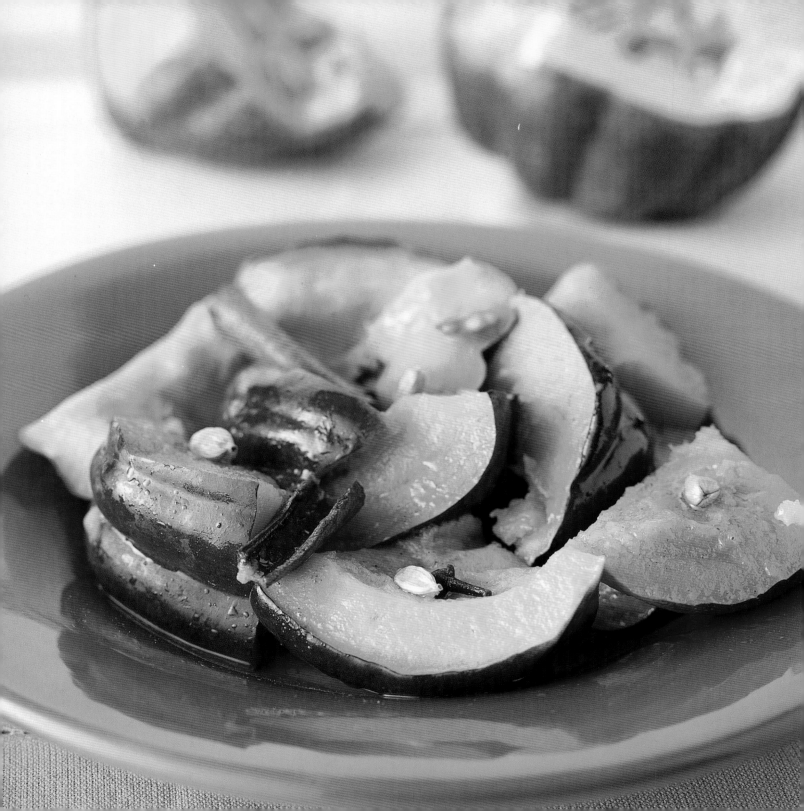

Vegetables & Salads

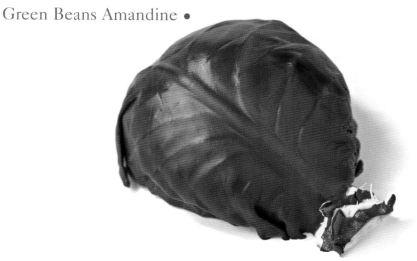

PREP TIME: 15 MINUTES   COOK TIME: 30 MINUTES
(REFRIGERATE 2 HOURS)

Mediterranean Eggplant Salad

MAKES 8 SERVINGS

A fast and interesting salad.

1/2 cup long-grain brown rice

1 medium eggplant

2 tablespoons vegetable oil

1 teaspoon salt

1 teaspoon ground cumin

1 teaspoon ground cinnamon

1 cup celery, thinly sliced

1/2 cup green onions, thinly sliced

8 large lettuce leaves

2 tomatoes

8 ounces lemon-flavored yogurt

● Prepare the rice as directed on package. Wash the eggplant and remove stem. Cut into 1-inch cubes. Heat the oil in a large skillet. Add eggplant and cook, stirring, until eggplant starts to brown. Add a small amount of water, cover tightly, and reduce heat. Uncover pan at short intervals and stir, adding extra water, if needed. Cook until eggplant is tender. Drain off any excess liquid. Remove from pan and stir in the salt, cumin, and cinnamon. Carefully stir in the rice. Cool to room temperature. Add celery and green onions. Place in bowl, cover, and refrigerate until completely chilled, about 2 hours or overnight. Place the lettuce leaves on 8 chilled salad plates. Divide salad equally among plates. Cut tomatoes into eighths; garnish each salad with 2 tomato wedges. Top with equal amounts of yogurt.

EACH SERVING: ABOUT 128 CALORIES, 4 G PROTEIN, 20 G CARBOHYDRATE,
4 G TOTAL FAT (1 G SATURATED), 1 MG CHOLESTEROL, 328 MG SODIUM.
EXCHANGE, 1 SERVING: 1 BREAD, 1 FAT

Best of Turnips

MAKES 6 SERVINGS

This is an easy and very flavorful recipe.

2 slices bacon
2 pounds fresh turnips

● In a large skillet, fry bacon until crisp; remove bacon from pan and crumble. Meanwhile, peel and finely grate the turnips. Place grated turnips in hot bacon fat. Toss and cook until turnips are well coated and slightly brown. Reduce heat; add a small amount of water to pan and cover tightly. Simmer on low heat until turnips are tender, about 15 to 20 minutes. Drain off any remaining water or fat. Stir in crumbled bacon. Serve hot.

EACH SERVING: ABOUT 113 CALORIES, 3 G PROTEIN, 9 G CARBOHYDRATE, 7 G TOTAL FAT (3 G SATURATED), 9 MG CHOLESTEROL, 194 MG SODIUM. EXCHANGE, 1 SERVING: 1 VEGETABLE, 1/2 FAT

Baked Red Onions

MAKES 4 SERVINGS

So easy to prepare, this vegetable dish features red onions—try it!

2 large red onions
1 tablespoon red wine vinegar
3 tablespoons water
2 teaspoons granulated sugar replacement
1/2 teaspoon salt
1/4 teaspoon ground sage
1/4 teaspoon dry mustard
2 tablespoons margarine

● Peel and cut onions in half crosswise. Place side by side, cut side up, in a shallow 8-inch baking pan. In a small bowl, blend together the vinegar, water, sugar replacement, salt, sage, and mustard. Pour over onion halves. Cover tightly. Bake at 350°F for 50 to 60 minutes or until onions are tender.

● Microwave: Reduce amount of water to 2 tablespoons. Cook on high for 5 to 10 minutes, turning dish every 3 minutes.

EACH SERVING: ABOUT 74 CALORIES, 1 G PROTEIN, 5 G CARBOHYDRATE, 6 G TOTAL FAT (1 G SATURATED), 0 MG CHOLESTEROL, 367 MG SODIUM. EXCHANGE, 1 SERVING: 1 VEGETABLE

Salade Niçoise

MAKES 4 SERVINGS

1/2 cup red wine vinegar salad dressing

1/2 cup Italian salad dressing

1/2 teaspoon dried dill

1/2 teaspoon oregano

dash black pepper

1/2 red or yellow onion, thinly sliced

3 ounces artichoke hearts, marinated and drained

1 cup fresh green beans, cut and trimmed, or frozen
   French-style green beans, thawed and drained

2 small heads Boston lettuce, torn into bite-size pieces

1/2 cucumber, sliced

2 tomatoes, cut into wedges

1/2 cup mushrooms, sliced

1/4 cup radishes, sliced

1/2 cup red pepper, sliced in thin strips

1 medium potato, cooked and sliced

1 7-ounce can tuna, packed in water, rinsed

1/4 cup pitted black olives, sliced

1 hard-cooked egg, chopped

● Combine salad dressings with dill, oregano, and pepper. Marinate onion, artichoke hearts, and green beans in dressing mixture for 2 to 3 hours. Before serving, combine the marinated vegetables and dressing with the remaining ingredients except the hard-cooked egg. Toss to mix well. Garnish with the chopped egg.

EACH SERVING: ABOUT 223 CALORIES, 18 G PROTEIN, 20 G CARBOHYDRATE, 9 G TOTAL FAT (2 G SATURATED), 72 MG CHOLESTEROL, 347 MG SODIUM. EXCHANGE, 1 SERVING: 2 LEAN MEAT, 3 VEGETABLES

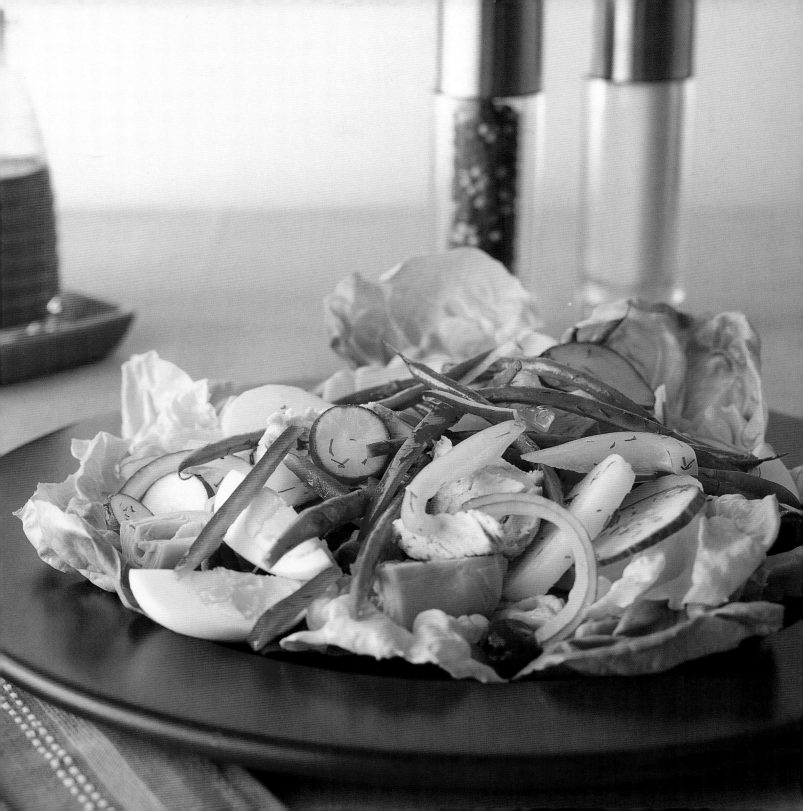

PREP TIME: 15 MINUTES   (MARINATE OVERNIGHT)

Mushroom & Watercress Salad

MAKES 8 SERVINGS

This is a delightful new taste for most people.

3 *cups snow-white mushrooms, medium size*

2 *tablespoons fresh lemon juice*

2 *tablespoons white wine vinegar*

2 *tablespoons olive oil*

1/3 *cup water*

1/2 *teaspoon salt*

1/2 *teaspoon dried tarragon, crushed*

1/4 *teaspoon ground basil*

1 *cup fresh watercress, chopped*

● Clean and slice mushrooms; place in a medium bowl. Mix together the lemon juice, vinegar, oil, water, salt, tarragon, and basil. Pour dressing over mushrooms, mixing carefully to completely coat the mushrooms. Marinate overnight in the refrigerator. Just before serving, drain extra dressing from mushrooms, add watercress, and toss to completely mix. Divide among 8 chilled salad plates.

EACH SERVING: ABOUT 39 CALORIES, 1 G PROTEIN, 2 G CARBOHYDRATE, 4 G TOTAL FAT (1 G SATURATED), 0 MG CHOLESTEROL, 147 MG SODIUM. EXCHANGE, 1 SERVING: 1/2 VEGETABLE, 1 FAT

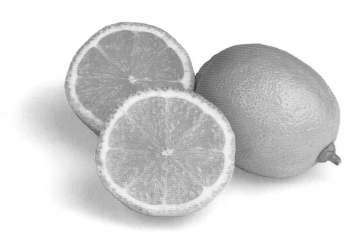

PREP TIME: 5 MINUTES   COOK TIME: 10 MINUTES

Pea Pods & Carrots

MAKES 4 SERVINGS

1 cup pea pods

1 cup carrots, sliced

1 teaspoon salt

2 teaspoons margarine

1 tablespoon Worcestershire sauce

● Combine pea pods and carrots in saucepan. Cover with water; add salt. Cook until tender; drain. Melt margarine in saucepan. Add Worcestershire sauce; stir to blend. Add pea pods and carrots. Toss to coat.

EACH SERVING: ABOUT 44 CALORIES, 1 G PROTEIN, 5 G CARBOHYDRATE, 2 G TOTAL FAT (TRACE SATURATED), 0 MG CHOLESTEROL, 268 MG SODIUM. EXCHANGE, 1 SERVING: 1/2 BREAD, 1/2 FAT

PREP TIME: 5 MINUTES   COOK TIME: 25 MINUTES

Zucchini Patties

MAKES 12 SMALL PATTIES (6-SERVINGS)

1/3 cup wheat germ

1/3 cup all-purpose flour

1/4 cup Parmesan cheese, grated

1/4 teaspoon baking powder

1/4 teaspoon oregano, crushed

dash salt

2 cups zucchini (about 2 medium), shredded

2 eggs, slightly beaten

● Combine wheat germ, flour, cheese, baking powder, oregano, and salt in a bowl. Stir well to blend. Add zucchini and eggs. Stir just to blend. Preheat griddle to 350°F. It is ready when drops of water skitter on the surface. Grease hot griddle for the first patties. Drop batter by spoonfuls onto griddle, spreading to flatten slightly. Bake until golden brown, about 3 to 4 minutes. Turn and bake on other side about 3 to 4 minutes. Continue making patties. Serve with favorite main dish, if desired.

EACH SERVING: ABOUT 95 CALORIES, 7 G PROTEIN, 10 G CARBOHYDRATE, 4 G TOTAL FAT (1 G SATURATED), 74 MG CHOLESTEROL, 105 MG SODIUM. EXCHANGE, 2 PATTIES: 2 VEGETABLES, 1/2 FAT

PREP TIME: 5 MINUTES   COOK TIME: 15 MINUTES

Crumb-Topped Zucchini and Tomatoes

MAKES 6 SERVINGS

3/4 cup bran flakes

2 teaspoons and 2 tablespoons margarine

1/2 teaspoon grated lemon peel

3 cups zucchini, cut in 1/4-inch slices

2 tablespoons margarine

1/4 teaspoon salt

dash pepper

1 tablespoon lemon juice

3 tomatoes, cut into wedges

• Crush cereal to make crumbs. Melt the 2 teaspoons margarine in small skillet. Stir in cereal crumbs. Cook over low heat, stirring constantly, until lightly browned. Remove from heat. Stir in lemon peel. Set aside for topping.

• In large skillet, cook zucchini in the 2 tablespoons margarine until almost tender, stirring frequently. Sprinkle with salt and pepper. Stir in lemon juice and tomato wedges. Continue cooking until tomatoes are heated. Spoon vegetable mixture into serving bowl. Top with cereal mixture. Serve immediately.

EACH SERVING: ABOUT 83 CALORIES, 2 G PROTEIN, 9 G CARBOHYDRATE, 6 G TOTAL FAT (1 G SATURATED), 0 MG CHOLESTEROL, 208 MG SODIUM. EXCHANGE, 1 SERVING: 2 VEGETABLES, 1 FAT

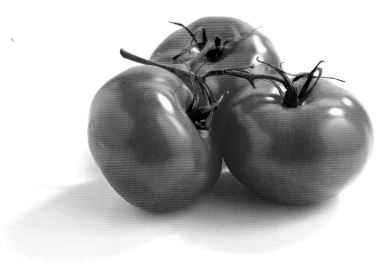

Cauliflower au Gratin

MAKES 4 SERVINGS

1 10-ounce package frozen cauliflower, thawed

Sauce

1 tablespoon butter

1 tablespoon all-purpose flour

1/4 teaspoon salt

dash pepper

1 teaspoon dry mustard

3/4 cup skim milk

1/2 cup Cheddar cheese, grated

Topping

1/4 cup wheat germ

1/4 cup bran flakes

2 teaspoons butter, melted

1/4 teaspoon dried sage

dash dry mustard

dash salt

● Spread cauliflower in bottom of ungreased 1-quart casserole. To prepare cheese sauce, melt butter in a saucepan and blend in flour and seasonings; stir until smooth. Remove from heat and stir in milk. Heat to boiling, stirring constantly. Add grated cheese and stir until melted and mixture is thickened. Pour sauce over cauliflower.

● Combine the topping ingredients and sprinkle over the sauce. Bake uncovered at 325°F for 15 minutes or until cauliflower is heated through and crisp-tender.

● Microwave: Combine ingredients as above. Cook on Medium for 3 minutes; turn and cook 2 minutes longer.

EACH SERVING: ABOUT 143 CALORIES, 7 G PROTEIN, 11 G CARBOHYDRATE, 9 G TOTAL FAT (5 G SATURATED), 23 MG CHOLESTEROL, 272 MG SODIUM. EXCHANGE, 1 SERVING: 2 VEGETABLE, 1 FAT

Asparagus to Perfection

MAKES 4 SERVINGS

This is especially great in the springtime when asparagus are in season.

1 pound fresh asparagus

8 ounces fresh mushrooms

1 tablespoon butter

1/2 teaspoon salt

1 teaspoon soy sauce

1/2 cup water

1/2 teaspoon cornstarch

● Wash asparagus and break off and discard the woody parts. Place spears on cutting board and slice diagonally into thin slices. Clean and slice mushrooms. Melt butter in a skillet; add asparagus and mushrooms. Stir to coat. Add salt and soy sauce; cook, stirring, for 4 minutes. Combine water and cornstarch in bowl or shaker jar. Blend completely. Add to asparagus. Cook until cornstarch mixture clears and slightly thickens.

EACH SERVING: ABOUT 68 CALORIES, 4 G PROTEIN, 8 G CARBOHYDRATE, 3 G TOTAL FAT (2 G SATURATED), 8 MG CHOLESTEROL, 408 MG SODIUM. EXCHANGE, 1 SERVING: 1 VEGETABLE, 1 FAT

Corn Pudding

MAKES 6 SERVINGS

1 16-ounce can corn

1 egg, beaten

1 teaspoon pimiento, chopped

1 teaspoon chopped green pepper

1 teaspoon margarine, melted

1 teaspoon sugar replacement

3/4 cup milk

salt and pepper to taste

vegetable cooking spray

● Combine all ingredients, except vegetable cooking spray. Pour into baking dish coated with vegetable cooking spray. Bake at 325°F for 35 to 40 minutes, or until firm.

EACH SERVING: ABOUT 89 CALORIES, 4 G PROTEIN, 16 G CARBOHYDRATE, 2 G TOTAL FAT (1 G SATURATED), 36 MG CHOLESTEROL 241 MG SODIUM. EXCHANGE, 1 SERVING: 1 BREAD, 1 FAT

Corn Pudding

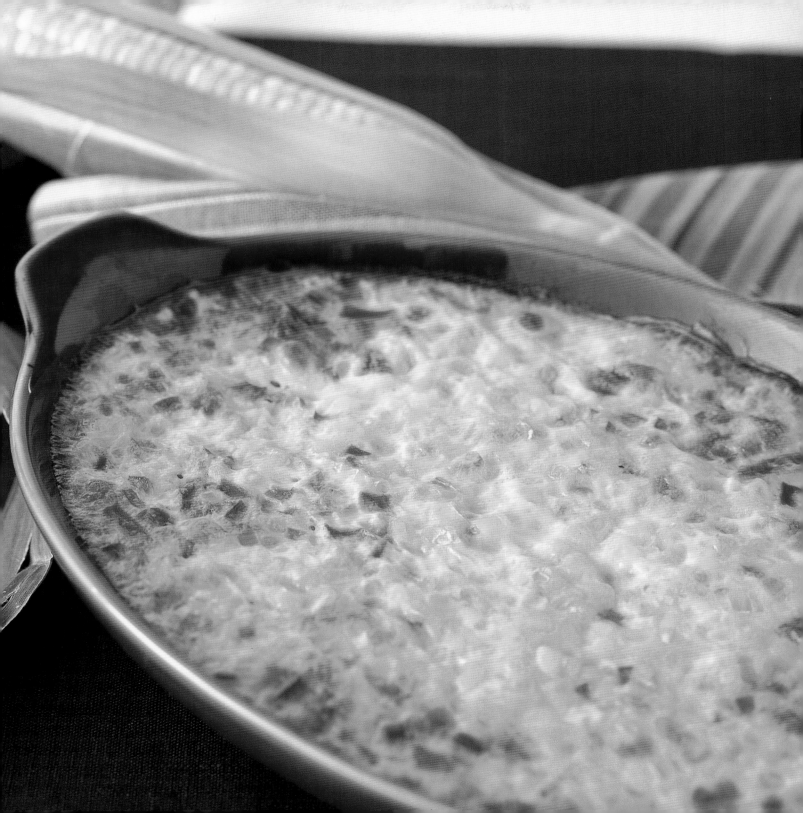

PREP TIME: 20 MINUTES   COOK TIME: 40 MINUTES

Tomato-Potato Salad

MAKES 8 SERVINGS

1 package au gratin potatoes

3³/4 cups water

1 package cheese-sauce mix

¹/3 cup low-calorie salad dressing

1 teaspoon prepared yellow mustard

2 eggs, hard-cooked

¹/2 cup coarsely chopped celery

8 tomatoes

• Combine dry potato slices and 3 cups water in a medium saucepan. Heat to boiling; then reduce heat and simmer, covered, for 15 to 20 minutes or until potatoes are just fork-tender. Rinse immediately with cold water. Drain well; then cover and chill thoroughly. In a small saucepan, combine the remaining ³/4 cup water and the package of dry cheese-sauce mix. Cook over medium heat while stirring, until mixture boils and thickens. Remove from heat and chill. To serve: Combine chilled cheese sauce, salad dressing, and mustard. Stir to blend thoroughly. Peel hard-cooked eggs and slice into chilled potatoes. Add celery to potatoes and fold in gently. Then fold in salad-dressing mixture. With the stem side down, cut tomatoes into eight wedges. Do not cut through the base of the tomato. Spread wedges apart slightly. Fill with salad. You can also make the filling beforehand and stuff the tomatoes when needed.

EACH SERVING: ABOUT 150 CALORIES, 6 G PROTEIN, 22 G CARBOHYDRATE, 6 G TOTAL FAT (3 G SATURATED), 62 MG CHOLESTEROL, 685 MG SODIUM. EXCHANGE, 1 SERVING: 1 STARCH/BREAD, 1 FAT

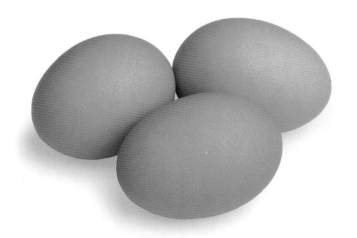

PREP TIME: 5 MINUTES   COOK TIME: 15 MINUTES

Green Beans Amandine

MAKES 4 SERVINGS

1 16-ounce can green beans, French style
2 tablespoons low-calorie margarine
1/4 cup slivered almonds
salt and pepper to taste

• Drain beans. Melt margarine in skillet. Add almonds and sauté until lightly browned. Add beans and warm thoroughly. Next, add salt and pepper to taste.

EACH SERVING: ABOUT 63 CALORIES, 2 G PROTEIN, 4 G CARBOHYDRATE, 5 G TOTAL FAT (1 G SATURATED), 0 MG CHOLESTEROL, 244 MG SODIUM. EXCHANGE, 1 SERVING: 1 VEGETABLE, 1/2 FAT

PREP TIME: 15 MINUTES   COOK TIME: 50 MINUTES

Cheesy Zucchini

MAKES 6 SERVINGS

1 pound zucchini
2 tablespoons low-calorie margarine
1 white onion, chopped
1 clove garlic, minced
1 pound tomatoes
2 tablespoons chopped fresh parsley
3/4 cup shredded Cheddar cheese
black pepper

• Wash and cut zucchini into 2-inch slices. Melt margarine in a skillet. Sauté onion and garlic in the margarine until transparent. Add zucchini and sauté for 5 minutes or until zucchini is almost tender. Peel and chop tomatoes. Add parsley to tomatoes and toss to incorporate. In the bottom of a lightly greased baking dish, place a layer of tomatoes; then add a layer of zucchini. Sprinkle with half the shredded Cheddar cheese and a small amount of black pepper. Finish with a layer of tomatoes, a layer of zucchini, and a layer of cheese. Bake at 350°F for 40 to 45 minutes.

EACH SERVING: ABOUT 137 CALORIES, 5 G PROTEIN, 9 G CARBOHYDRATE, 9 G TOTAL FAT (4 G SATURATED), 15 MG CHOLESTEROL, 258 MG SODIUM. EXCHANGE, 1 SERVING: 1 VEGETABLE, 1 FAT

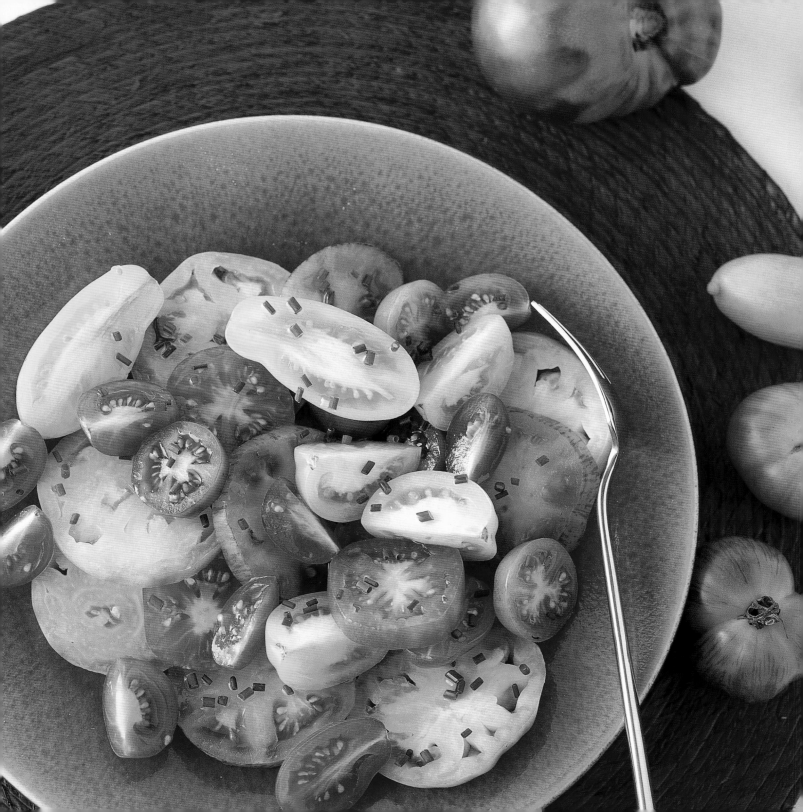

PREP TIME: 5 MINUTES

Tomatoes Vinaigrette

MAKES 4 SERVINGS

Vary the color and type of tomatoes used in this dish to create a beautiful array of colors and shapes.

2 large tomatoes, unpeeled and thinly sliced
2 tablespoons water
1 tablespoon vegetable oil
1 tablespoon red wine vinegar
1/4 teaspoon salt
dash dried basil
dash black pepper
2 tablespoons chives, chopped

● Arrange tomato slices on 4 serving plates. Combine water, oil, vinegar, salt, basil, and pepper in a bowl or jar. Stir to completely blend. Sprinkle tomato slices with dressing. Garnish with chives.

EACH SERVING: ABOUT 44 CALORIES, 1 G PROTEIN, 3 G CARBOHYDRATE, 4 G TOTAL FAT (1 G SATURATED), 0 MG CHOLESTEROL, 150 MG SODIUM. EXCHANGE, 1 SERVING: 1/2 VEGETABLE, 1/2 FAT

PREP TIME: 20 MINUTES   COOK TIME: 20 TO 30 MINUTES

Heavenly Eggplant Slices

MAKES 6 SERVINGS

1 large eggplant
2 tablespoons vegetable oil
3 tomatoes, cored and cubed
1 medium yellow onion, finely chopped
1 teaspoon granulated sugar replacement
1 teaspoon gingerroot, finely chopped
1/4 teaspoon ground ginger
1/4 teaspoon salt
dash pepper
3 tablespoons fresh parsley, chopped

● Slice unpeeled eggplant in 1-inch slices. Brush oil on both sides of slices. Arrange in single layer in a baking dish. Place tomatoes in blender; blend to a purée. In a large saucepan, combine tomato pureé, onion, sugar replacement, gingerroot, ground ginger, salt, and pepper. Cook and stir over medium heat until onions are translucent. Pour sauce over eggplant slices. Bake at 400°F for 20 to 30 minutes or until eggplant is tender. Garnish with parsley.

EACH SERVING: ABOUT 68 CALORIES, 4 G PROTEIN, 8 G CARBOHYDRATE, 3 G TOTAL FAT (2 G SATURATED), 8 MG CHOLESTEROL, 408 MG SODIUM. EXCHANGE, 1 SERVING: 1/2 VEGETABLE, 1 FAT

Tomatoes Vinaigrette

Stir-Fried Vegetables

MAKES 6 SERVINGS

2 tablespoons olive oil

1 small piece ginger, grated

1/2 cup chopped onion

1 green pepper, cut in strips

1 red pepper, cut in strips

1/2 cup celery, sliced

1/2 cup carrots, sliced

1 cup broccoli florets

1 cup sliced mushrooms

1 tablespoon soy sauce

● Heat the olive oil in a wok. Add grated ginger and fry for 1 minute. Remove ginger from wok. Add onion, green and red peppers, celery, and carrots. Fry for 3 minutes, tossing vegetables as they fry. Add broccoli and mushrooms. Toss vegetables. Add small amount of water. Cover and allow to simmer for 2 to 3 minutes. Next, add soy sauce. Fry without cover for 1 minute. Serve in wok, or transfer to heated plate or dish.

EACH SERVING: ABOUT 69 CALORIES, 2 G PROTEIN, 7 G CARBOHYDRATE, 5 G TOTAL FAT (1 G SATURATED), 0 MG CHOLESTEROL, 189 MG SODIUM. EXCHANGE, 1 SERVING: 1 VEGETABLE, 1 FAT

Spinach with Onion

MAKES 4 SERVINGS

2 pounds fresh spinach

2 teaspoons margarine

1/2 cup onion, sliced

dash nutmeg

dash thyme

salt and pepper to taste

● Rinse spinach thoroughly; place in top of double boiler and heat until wilted. Drain and chop coarsely. Melt margarine in skillet; add onion. Sauté over high heat until onion is brown on the edges. Add seasonings. Stir to blend. Add spinach and toss to blend.

EACH SERVING: ABOUT 77 CALORIES, 7 G PROTEIN, 10 G CARBOHYDRATE, 3 G TOTAL FAT (0 G SATURATED), 0 MG CHOLESTEROL, 180 MG SODIUM. EXCHANGE, 1 SERVING: 1/2 VEGETABLE, 1/2 FAT

PREP TIME: 5 MINUTES   COOK TIME: 55 MINUTES

Zucchini Florentine

MAKES 6 SERVINGS

4 small zucchini

2 teaspoons margarine

1 cup fresh spinach, chopped

1 cup skim milk

3 eggs, slightly beaten

1 teaspoon salt

1/4 teaspoon pepper

1/4 teaspoon thyme

1/4 teaspoon paprika

• Cut zucchini into thin slices. Melt margarine in baking dish; add zucchini. Bake at 400°F for 15 minutes. Add spinach. Blend skim milk, eggs, salt, pepper, and thyme. Pour over vegetables. Sprinkle with paprika. Bake at 350°F for 40 minutes, or until set.

EACH SERVING: ABOUT 78 CALORIES, 6 G PROTEIN, 5 G CARBOHYDRATE, 4 G TOTAL FAT (1 G SATURATED), 108 MG CHOLESTEROL, 461 MG SODIUM. EXCHANGE, 1 SERVING: 1 VEGETABLE, 1/2 HIGH-FAT MEAT

PREP TIME: 15 MINUTE   (REFRIGERATE 2 HOURS)

Herbed Cottage Cheese Salad

MAKES 8 SERVINGS

1 16-ounce container low-calorie cottage cheese

1/2 cup low-calorie sour cream

1/2 cup cucumber, peeled, seeded, and chopped

1/3 cup green pepper, chopped

1 tablespoon chives, chopped

pinch tarragon

pinch summer savory

pinch dill seed

8 leaves iceberg lettuce

• Combine cottage cheese, sour cream, cucumber, green pepper, herbs, and dill seed in a bowl. Stir to mix. Cover and refrigerate for at least 2 hours. Arrange lettuce leaves on eight plates. Scoop cottage-cheese salad in middle of each leaf.

EACH SERVING: ABOUT 65 CALORIES, 8 G PROTEIN, 3 G CARBOHYDRATE, 2 G TOTAL FAT (2 G SATURATED), 8 MG CHOLESTEROL, 237 MG SODIUM. EXCHANGE, EACH SERVING: 1 LOW-FAT MILK, 1/2 FAT

PREP TIME: 5 MINUTES   COOK TIME: 10 MINUTES

Sautéed Cherry Tomatoes

MAKES 1 SERVING

2 teaspoons olive oil

1 clove garlic, sliced

1 cup cherry tomatoes, rinsed

dash salt

dash pepper

dash basil

● Heat oil in small skillet. Add garlic and cherry tomatoes. Heat by tilting the pan so that the tomatoes roll. Cherry tomatoes cook and burst quickly. Do not overcook. Just as the tomatoes are showing signs of softening, sprinkle with salt, pepper, and basil. Serve immediately. (If you are making a larger quantity than the recipe calls for, cook in a large heavy pan. Do not crowd the tomatoes or prevent them from rolling.)

EACH SERVING: ABOUT 115 CALORIES, 2 G PROTEIN, 8 G CARBOHYDRATE, 9 G TOTAL FAT (1 G SATURATED), 0 MG CHOLESTEROL, 14 MG SODIUM. EXCHANGE: 1 VEGETABLE, 2 FAT

PREP TIME: 5 MINUTES   COOK TIME: 20 MINUTES

Indian Squash

MAKES 4 SERVINGS

2 cups acorn squash, cubed

2 teaspoons margarine

1 teaspoon grated orange rind

1/4 cup orange juice

2 tablespoons sugar replacement

● Cook squash in small amount of boiling water until crisp-tender; drain. Melt margarine in saucepan. Add orange rind, juice, and sugar replacement. Cook over low heat until sugar is dissolved. Add squash; cover and continue cooking until squash is tender.

EACH SERVING: ABOUT 52 CALORIES, 1 G PROTEIN, 9 G CARBOHYDRATE, 2 G TOTAL FAT (TRACE SATURATED), 0 MG CHOLESTEROL, 28 MG SODIUM. EXCHANGE, 1 SERVING: 1 BREAD, 1/2 FAT

Indian Squash

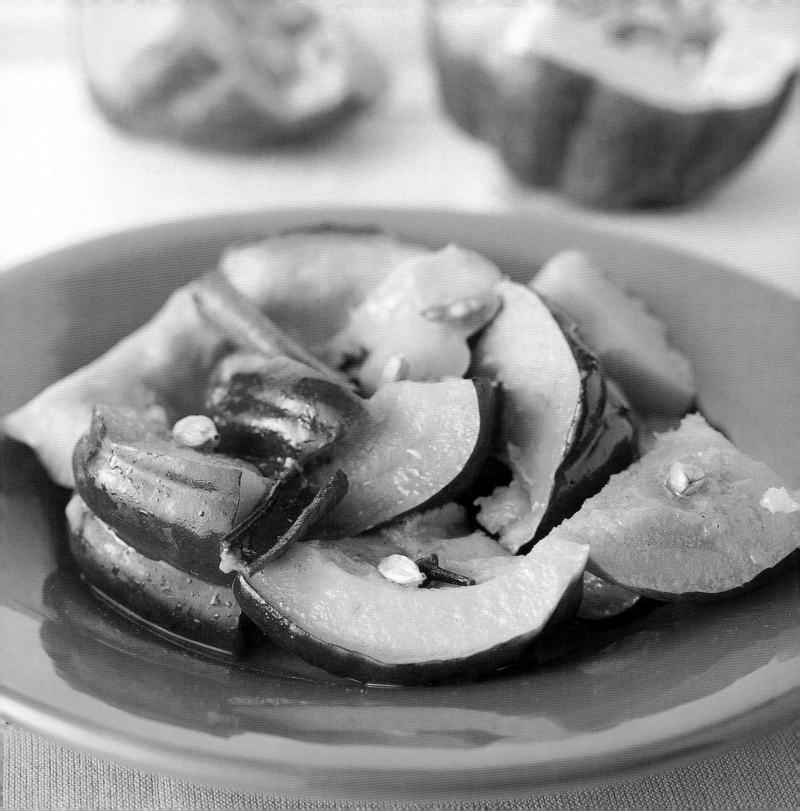

PREP TIME: 15 MINUTES   COOK TIME: 10 MINUTES

Brussels Sprouts with Butter Crumbs

MAKES 4 SERVINGS

1 pound Brussels sprouts, rinsed and trimmed

3 tablespoons low-calorie margarine

1/3 cup dry bread crumbs

1 envelope natural butter-flavored mix

1 tablespoon lemon juice

freshly ground black pepper

● Cook Brussels sprouts in boiling water for about 15 minutes or until tender. Drain and transfer to heated baking dish. Keep warm. Melt margarine in small skillet; then add bread crumbs and sauté until golden brown. Sprinkle bread crumbs with butter mix. Toss to coat completely. Stir in lemon juice. Pour over Brussels sprouts. Sprinkle with black pepper.

EACH SERVING: ABOUT 123 CALORIES, 5 G PROTEIN, 17 G CARBOHYDRATE, 5 G TOTAL FAT (1 G SATURATED), 0 MG CHOLESTEROL, 210 MG SODIUM. EXCHANGE, EACH SERVING: 1 VEGETABLE, 1 FAT, 1/2 STARCH/BREAD

PREP TIME: 20 MINUTES   COOK TIME: 10 MINUTES

Leeks and Mushrooms

MAKES 3 SERVINGS

1 pound small mushrooms

6 leeks

1/2 red pepper

2 tablespoons low-calorie margarine

salt and pepper to taste

● Clean mushrooms and remove stems. Thinly slice the white part of the leeks. Slice the red pepper in thin strips. Melt the margarine in a saucepan over low heat. Add vegetables, salt, and pepper. Cover tightly. Allow to cook over low heat for 2 minutes. Remove lid and toss vegetables. Replace lid on saucepan and cook for 2 more minutes. Remove lid and cook over high heat to evaporate any liquid. Transfer to heated plate or chafing dish.

EACH SERVING: ABOUT 185 CALORIES, 7 G PROTEIN, 33 G CARBOHYDRATE, 5 G TOTAL FAT (1 G SATURATED), 0 MG CHOLESTEROL, 135 MG SODIUM. EXCHANGE, EACH SERVING: 1/2 VEGETABLE, 1 FAT

South of the Border Salad Tray

MAKES 12 SERVINGS

This is a grand version of Pico de Gallo ("beak of the rooster") relish.

2 *medium cucumbers*
1/2 cup cider vinegar
2 *tablespoons vegetable oil*
1 *teaspoon salt*
1 *large white onion*
3 *large oranges*
1 *tablespoon lemon juice*
1/2 cup cold water
1 *large avocado*
Bibb lettuce leaves
1/2 teaspoon red pepper

● With a vegetable parer, peel strips lengthwise from each cucumber to make alternating green and white stripes. Cut off the ends and thinly slice the cucumbers into rounds; place in a large bowl. Add vinegar, oil, and salt. Mix and chill for at least 2 hours. (This can be made a day in advance.) To arrange salad, lift cucumbers from marinade, and save the marinade. Drain slightly. Peel onion and oranges and thinly slice lengthwise. Combine lemon juice and water in a small bowl. Peel and thinly slice the avocado; drop avocado slices into the lemon water to avoid discoloration. On a large platter or tray, arrange separate sections of cucumber, onion, orange, and avocado slices. Garnish with lettuce leaves. Just before serving, combine reserved cucumber marinade with the red pepper. Pour over entire salad.

EACH SERVING: ABOUT 73 CALORIES, 1 G PROTEIN, 8 G CARBOHYDRATE, 5 G TOTAL FAT (1 G SATURATED), 0 MG CHOLESTEROL, 196 MG SODIUM. EXCHANGE, EACH SERVING: 1/2 FRUIT, 1 FAT

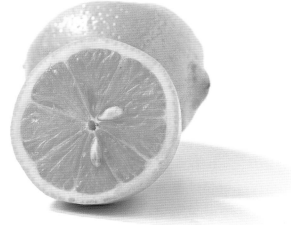

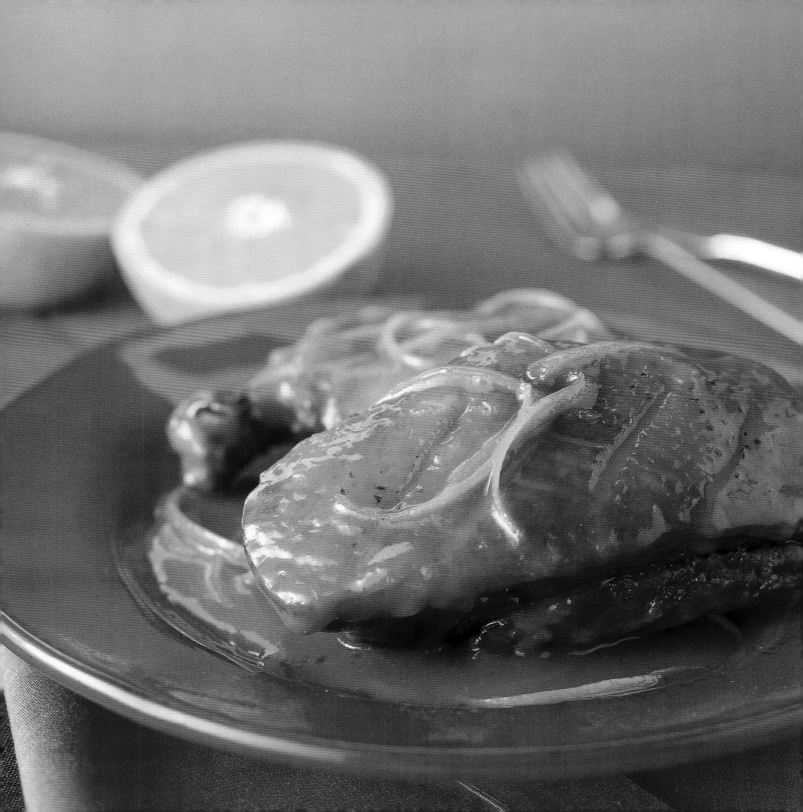

Chicken & Poultry

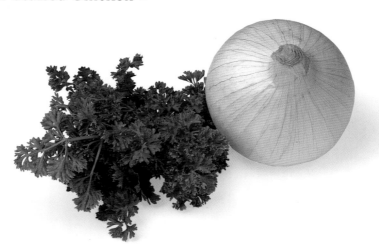

Chicken and Corn Hot Dish

MAKES 6 SERVINGS

1 tablespoon butter

1 cup fresh mushrooms, sliced

1 tablespoon flour

1 cup chicken broth

2 cups cooked chicken, diced

2 cups cooked whole kernel corn

2 cups cooked elbow macaroni

• Heat butter in large skillet; cook until lightly browned. Add mushrooms and sauté until tender. Remove mushrooms from skillet. Add flour to remaining butter in skillet and mix well. Stir in chicken broth and cook over low heat until mixture thickens, stirring constantly. Add chicken, corn, and macaroni. Stir to completely blend. Cook and stir over low heat until mixture is thoroughly heated.

EACH SERVING: ABOUT 231 CALORIES, 20 G PROTEIN, 28 G CARBOHYDRATE,
5 G TOTAL FAT (1 G SATURATED), 40 MG CHOLESTEROL, 124 MG SODIUM.
EXCHANGE, 1 SERVING: 1 BREAD, 2 VEGETABLE, 1 HIGH-FAT MEAT

El Dorado

MAKES 1 SERVING

1/2 cup chicken broth

1/2 ounce fresh oysters

1 teaspoon margarine

1 tablespoon grated carrot

2 tablespoons chopped celery

1 teaspoon chopped parsley

1 ounce cooked chicken, diced

salt and pepper to taste

• Heat chicken broth to a boil; add oysters. Cook until edges roll; reserve cooking liquid. Heat margarine in heavy skillet. Add carrot, celery, and parsley. Sauté until crisp-tender. Add chicken, oysters, and 1 tablespoon of the chicken broth. Cook until thoroughly heated. Drain, if necessary. Add salt and pepper.

EACH SERVING: ABOUT 120 CALORIES, 12 G PROTEIN, 3 G CARBOHYDRATE,
6 G TOTAL FAT (1 G SATURATED), 28 MG CHOLESTEROL, 450 MG SODIUM.
EXCHANGE: 1 1/2 LEAN MEAT, 2 FAT

Bran Parmesan Chicken

MAKES 4 SERVINGS

1¹/2 cups bran flakes cereal

1 egg

¹/4 cup milk

¹/4 cup all-purpose flour

dash salt

dash pepper

¹/4 teaspoon ground sage

3 tablespoons Parmesan cheese, grated

16 ounces chicken, cut in pieces

1 tablespoon margarine, melted

● Crush enough cereal to measure ³/4 cup in a shallow dish. Lightly beat together the egg and milk. Add flour, salt, pepper, sage, and cheese, stirring until smooth. Dip chicken pieces in the egg mixture. Coat with crushed cereal. Place in a single layer, skin side up, in greased or foil-lined shallow baking pan. Drizzle with margarine. Bake, uncovered, at 350°F for about 45 minutes or until tender, without turning chicken while baking.

EACH SERVING: ABOUT 267 CALORIES, 32 G PROTEIN, 18 G CARBOHYDRATE, 7 G TOTAL FAT (2 G SATURATED), 122 MG CHOLESTEROL, 358 MG SODIUM. EXCHANGE, 1 SERVING: 1 BREAD, 3 LEAN MEAT, 1 FAT

Crispy Wheat Germ Chicken

MAKES 4 SERVINGS

1 cup wheat germ

1 teaspoon dried tarragon, crushed*

1 teaspoon lemon rind, grated*

¹/4 cup milk

3 pounds broiler-fryer chicken, cut up and skinned

● Combine wheat germ, tarragon, and lemon rind in a shallow container. Stir well to blend. Pour milk into another shallow container. Dip chicken pieces in milk, then in wheat germ mixture, coating evenly. Place on foil-lined 15¹/2" x 10¹/2" x 1" jelly roll pan. Bake, uncovered, at 375°F for 40 to 50 minutes until tender.

*One teaspoon crushed oregano and a dash of garlic powder may be used instead of the tarragon and lemon rind.

EACH SERVING: ABOUT 581 CALORIES, 75 G PROTEIN, 15 G CARBOHYDRATE, 23 G TOTAL FAT (6 G SATURATED), 276 MG CHOLESTEROL, 288 MG SODIUM. EXCHANGE, 1 SERVING: 1 BREAD, 5 LEAN MEAT

Festive Party Chicken

MAKES 24 SERVINGS

12 6-ounce chicken breasts

6 cups cooked long-grain rice

1 1/2 cups golden raisins

2 1/2 teaspoons salt

4 5-ounce cans chow mein noodles

6 tablespoons butter, melted

7 1/2 cups pineapple tidbits in their juice

4 cups mandarin oranges

1 1/2 tablespoons lemon juice

6 tablespoons cornstarch

6 tablespoons soy sauce

6 tablespoons butter, cut into bits

2 8-ounce cans water chestnuts, drained
   and sliced

● Cut chicken breasts in half, remove bones, and cut through thickest part of each piece to form a pocket. In a bowl, mix rice, raisins, salt, and chow mein noodles; stuff 1/2 cup of the mixture into each breast; fasten with toothpicks and tie with string. Place chicken in buttered shallow baking pans, and brush with melted butter; bake at 350°F for 30 minutes. In a heavy pan, drain juice from pineapples and oranges and blend with lemon juice, cornstarch, and soy sauce. Cook over medium heat, stirring constantly until sauce is thick and transparent. Remove from heat and add butter, pineapple, oranges, and water chestnuts; mix well. Spoon over chicken and cover with aluminum foil. Bake at 325°F for 30 minutes longer or until chicken is tender. Remove toothpicks and string. Serve sauce over chicken.

EACH SERVING: ABOUT 488 CALORIES, 32 G PROTEIN, 57 G CARBOHYDRATE,
15 G TOTAL FAT (4 G SATURATED), 80 MG CHOLESTEROL, 703 MG SODIUM.
EXCHANGE, 1 SERVING: 1 BREAD, 3 LEAN MEAT

PREP TIME: 30 MINUTES   COOK TIME: 30 MINUTES

Sweet and Sour Chicken Breast

MAKES 4 SERVINGS

The sweet touches of pineapple and cherries add flavor and fiber to this colorful entrée.

2 tablespoons margarine

4 4-ounce chicken breasts, boned

1 16-ounce can tart cherries

1 8-ounce can crushed pineapple in its own juice

1/4 cup dry sherry

2 tablespoons soy sauce

1 clove garlic, minced

1 tablespoon gingerroot, chopped

1 cup celery, sliced

1/2 cup sweet red pepper, cut in chunks

1 tablespoon cornstarch

1/4 cup water

● Melt margarine in a skillet and brown chicken breasts. Drain juices from cherries and pineapple into a mixing bowl. Reserve the fruit and add sherry, soy sauce, garlic, and ginger to the juices. Stir to blend. Pour juice mixture over chicken. Cover and simmer 30 minutes. Remove chicken to warm serving dish and keep hot. Combine cherries, pineapple, celery, and red pepper in the pan. Dissolve cornstarch in the water and stir into pan. Cook and stir until mixture thickens. Pour over chicken.

EACH SERVING: ABOUT 413 CALORIES, 56 G PROTEIN, 21 G CARBOHYDRATE, 9 G TOTAL FAT (2 G SATURATED), 137 MG CHOLESTEROL, 783 MG SODIUM. EXCHANGE, 1 SERVING: 2 FRUIT, 1 HIGH-FAT MEAT

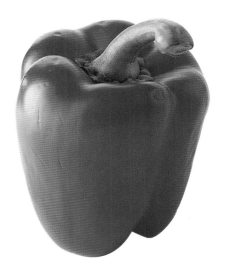

Pollo Lesso

MAKES 1 SERVING

1 3-ounce chicken breast, boned

1/2 tomato, quartered

1/4 cucumber, peeled and sliced

1/4 cup peas

dash salt

dash pepper

dash parsley

• Remove skin from chicken breast; boil chicken in small amount of salted water until almost tender. Add tomato pieces, cucumber slices, and peas. Heat thoroughly; drain. Place on serving plate. Sprinkle with salt, pepper, and parsley.

• Microwave: Place skinned chicken beast in individual dish; cover with plastic wrap. Cook on High for 12 minutes. Drain off any moisture. Add vegetables. Cook on Medium for 4 minutes. Sprinkle with salt, pepper, and parsley.

EACH SERVING: ABOUT 136 CALORIES, 23G PROTEIN, 8 G CARBOHYDRATE, 2 G TOTAL FAT (TRACE SATURATED), 49 MG CHOLESTEROL, 237 MG SODIUM. EXCHANGE: 3 LEAN MEAT, 1 BREAD

Scalloped Turkey and Cauliflower

MAKES 4 SERVINGS

2 cups fresh cauliflower florets

1 1/2 cups turkey stock

2 tablespoons whole wheat flour

1 teaspoon parsley flakes

2 teaspoons onion flakes

1 teaspoon salt

1/4 teaspoon black pepper

8 ounces cooked turkey breast

• Cook cauliflower in boiling, salted water for 6 minutes or until almost tender. Drain. Combine stock, flour, and seasonings in a small saucepan. Cook and stir until mixture is slightly thickened. Place turkey breast in a greased baking pan. Arrange cauliflower around turkey breast. Pour sauce over turkey and cauliflower. Bake in a 350°F oven for 20 to 25 minutes or until heated through.

EACH SERVING: ABOUT 231 CALORIES, 20 G PROTEIN, 28 G CARBOHYDRATE, 5 G TOTAL FAT (1 G SATURATED), 40 MG CHOLESTEROL, 124 MG SODIUM. EXCHANGE, 1 SERVING: 1 MEDIUM-FAT MEAT, 1 VEGETABLE

PREP TIME: 15 MINUTES   COOK TIME: 25 MINUTES

Turkey Divan

MAKES 4 SERVINGS

1 10-ounce package frozen broccoli spears

8 ounces unsalted, cooked turkey breast,
    thickly sliced

2 packages low-sodium mushroom soup mix

1/2 cup boiling water

1/2 cup skim milk

1/3 cup Cheddar cheese, shredded

• Cook broccoli until just tender as directed on package; drain. With stems towards the middle, arrange broccoli in a 1 1/2-quart casserole or round 9-inch baking dish. Place turkey slices in an even layer on top. Combine soup mix with 1/2 cup boiling water. Blend in milk and cheese. Pour sauce over turkey. Bake at 375°F for 25 minutes or until sauce begins to bubble.

EACH SERVING: ABOUT 283 CALORIES, 22 G PROTEIN, 25 G CARBOHYDRATE, 11 G FAT (2 G SATURATED), 27 MG CHOLESTEROL, 1,052 MG SODIUM. EXCHANGE, 1 SERVING: 2 1/2 LEAN MEAT, 1 VEGETABLE

PREP TIME: 5 MINUTES   COOK TIME: 15 MINUTES

Turkey à la King

MAKES 1 SERVING

1 tablespoon green pepper, diced

2 tablespoons celery, sliced

1/4 cup condensed cream of chicken soup

2 tablespoons skim milk

2 tablespoons mushrooms, chopped

3 ounces cooked turkey, diced

1 tablespoon pimiento, chopped

salt and pepper to taste

2 slices bread, toasted

• Cook green pepper and celery in boiling water until tender; drain. Blend condensed soup and skim milk. Add green pepper, celery, mushrooms, turkey, and pimiento. Add salt and pepper. Heat slightly over low heat. Cut toast into triangles; place in small bowl, tips ups. Spoon turkey mixture over tips.

EACH SERVING: ABOUT 325 CALORIES, 28 G PROTEIN, 34 G CARBOHYDRATE, 9 G TOTAL FAT (2 G SATURATED), 21 MG CHOLESTEROL, 1,158 MG SODIUM. EXCHANGE: 3 MEDIUM-FAT MEAT, 2 1/4 BREAD, 1/4 VEGETABLE

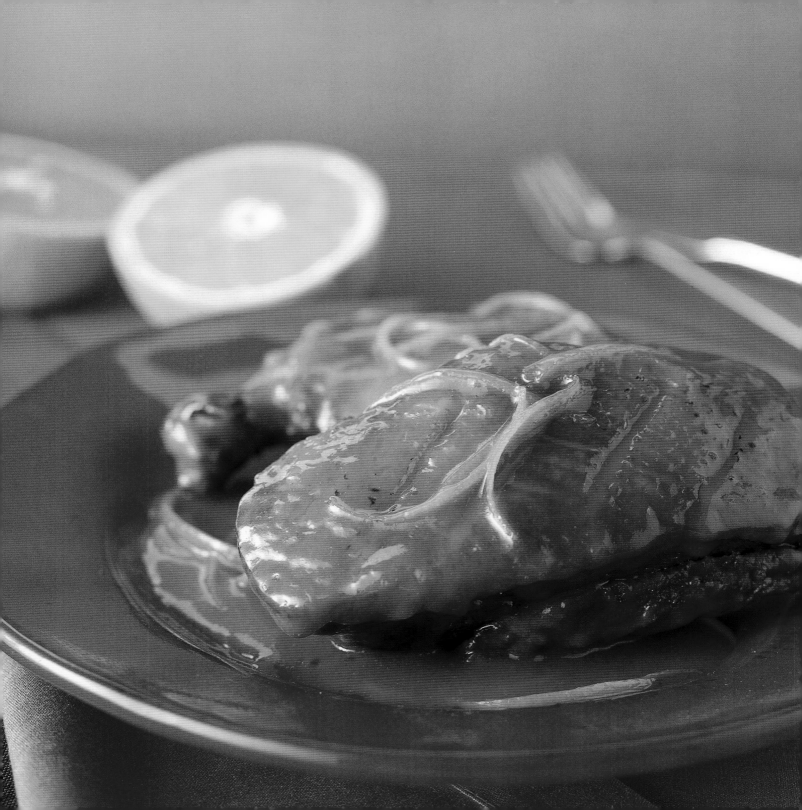

PREP TIME: 25 MINUTES   COOK TIME: 2 HOURS

Roast Duck with Orange Sauce

MAKES 64 APPETIZER SERVINGS

4- to 5-pound duck
salt to taste
2 medium oranges
Orange Sauce (below)

• Wash inside and outside of duck thoroughly. Remove any fat from tail or neck opening. Salt interior of bird. Cut each orange (with peel) into 8 sections. Place inside duck. Secure tail and neck skin, legs and wings with poultry pins. Salt exterior of duck. Place breast side up on a rack in roasting pan. Bake at 350°F for 2 hours. During the final hour, baste with Orange Sauce every 15 minutes.

EACH SERVING: ABOUT 117 CALORIES, 3 G PROTEIN, 1 G CARBOHYDRATE, 11 G TOTAL FAT (4 G SATURATED), 22 MG CHOLESTEROL, 18 MG SODIUM. EXCHANGE, EACH SERVING: 1 HIGH-FAT MEAT

Orange Sauce

MAKES 1/2 CUP

1/2 teaspoon cornstarch
2 tablespoons cold water
1/2 cup orange juice concentrate
2 teaspoons unsweetened orange drink mix

• Dissolve cornstarch in water. Add orange juice concentrate and drink mix. Cook over low heat until slightly thickened. Use as glaze on poultry or pork.

ABOUT 116 CALORIES, 1 G PROTEIN, 28 G CARBOHYDRATE, TRACE TOTAL FAT (0 G SATURATED), 0 MG CHOLESTEROL, 11 MG SODIUM. EXCHANGE: 1 FRUIT

Roast Duck with Orange Sauce

PREP TIME: 10 MINUTES

Chicken Cucumber Sandwiches

MAKES 8 SERVINGS

1 cup cooked chicken, diced
1/3 cup cucumber, peeled, seeded, and chopped
1/4 cup low-calorie blue-cheese salad dressing
1 cup lettuce, shredded

• Combine chicken, cucumber, and salad dressing in a bowl. Toss to mix. Fill sandwiches and then top with shredded lettuce. (This filling is excellent in pita pockets.)

EACH SERVING: ABOUT 69 CALORIES, 6 G PROTEIN, 1 G CARBOHYDRATE, 5 G TOTAL FAT (1 G SATURATED), 16 MG CHOLESTEROL, 16 MG SODIUM. EXCHANGE, 1 SERVING: 1 LEAN MEAT

PREP TIME: 20 MINUTES   COOK TIME: 2 HOURS 20 MINUTES

Giblet-Stuffed Chicken

MAKES 1 SERVING

2 giblets

1 teaspoon margarine

2 tablespoons rice

1 tablespoon raisins

1 tablespoon unsalted peanuts

salt and pepper to taste

1/4 cup water

3-ounce chicken breast, skinned and boned

• Simmer giblets in boiling water for 1 hour, or until tender. Drain. Remove tough center core from giblets. Chop giblets into small pieces. Melt margarine in small skillet. Sauté rice, raisins, giblets, and peanuts until rice and giblets are golden brown. Remove from heat. Add salt and pepper. Add 1/4 cup water. Cover and return to heat. Simmer for 15 minutes or until water is absorbed. Remove from heat. Remove cover and allow to cool slightly. Place chicken breast, boned side up, between two sheets of plastic wrap or waxed paper. Pound from center with the heel of your hand or edge of a plate to flatten. Place stuffing in center. Fold over and secure with toothpicks or poultry pins. Place in small baking dish. Bake in preheated oven at 350°F for 1 hour, or until golden brown.

• Microwave: Sprinkle with paprika and parsley. Cook on High for 18 minutes.

EACH SERVING: ABOUT 426 CALORIES, 50 G PROTEIN, 17 G CARBOHYDRATE, 17 G TOTAL FAT (4 G SATURATED), 442 MG CHOLESTEROL, 173 MG SODIUM. EXCHANGE: 3 1/2 LEAN MEAT, 1/2 FRUIT, 1/4 BREAD, 1 1/2 FAT

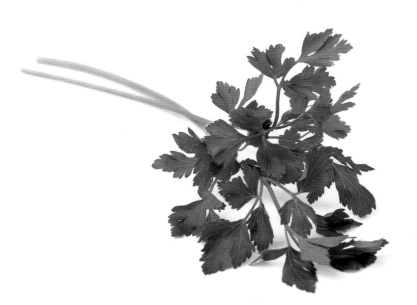

PREP TIME: 15 MINUTES

Soy Chicken Salad

MAKES 3 SERVINGS

A lovely salad to serve on a hot July day.

2 cups cooked chicken, shredded

1/2 cup cucumber, sliced

1/2 cup alfalfa sprouts

1 egg, hard-boiled and chopped

2 tablespoons lemon juice

1 tablespoon vegetable oil

2 teaspoons water

2 teaspoons soy sauce

1/2 teaspoon Dijon mustard

dash black pepper

● Combine chicken, cucumber, sprouts, and egg in a medium bowl. Cover tightly and refrigerate until serving time. To make the dressing, blend remaining ingredients. Just before serving, pour dressing over salad. Toss to completely coat the salad.

EACH SERVING: ABOUT 275 CALORIES, 35 G PROTEIN, 3 G CARBOHYDRATE, 13 G TOTAL FAT (3 G SATURATED), 272 MG CHOLESTEROL, 364 MG SODIUM. EXCHANGE, 1 SERVING: 2 LEAN MEAT, 1/2 VEGETABLE

PREP TIME: 10 MINUTES   COOK TIME: 30 MINUTES

Crafty Chicken

MAKES 1 SERVING

2 ounces chicken breast, boned

1 tablespoon all-purpose flour

salt and pepper to taste

1/2 strip bacon

● Remove skin from chicken breast. Combine flour, salt, and pepper in a bowl or on a piece of waxed paper. Stir to mix. Roll chicken breast in flour mixture. Place chicken breast in baking dish. Lay the 1/2 strip of bacon on top of chicken breast. Add 1/2 inch of water. Bake at 350°F for 30 minutes or until chicken is tender.

ABOUT 154 CALORIES, 15 G PROTEIN, 6 G CARBOHYDRATE, 7 G TOTAL FAT (3 G SATURATED), 41 MG CHOLESTEROL, 120 MG SODIUM. EXCHANGE: 2 LEAN MEAT

PREP TIME: 10 MINUTES

Chicken Delight

MAKES 1 SERVING

1/4 cup cooked chicken, finely chopped

1 tablespoon green pepper, finely chopped

1 tablespoon onion, finely chopped

1/4 teaspoon poultry seasoning

● Combine chicken, green pepper, onion, and poultry seasoning in a bowl. With a spoon, stir to make mixture sticky. If needed, add 1 or 2 drops of water.

ABOUT 65 CALORIES, 11 G PROTEIN, 2 G CARBOHYDRATE,
1 G TOTAL FAT (1 G SATURATED), 30 MG CHOLESTEROL, 27 MG SODIUM.
EXCHANGE: 1 LEAN MEAT

PREP TIME: 10 MINUTES   COOK TIME: 20 MINUTES

Sweet and Sour Chicken with Rice

MAKES 2 SERVINGS

1/4 cup crushed pineapple, in its own juice

2 teaspoons vinegar

1/2 teaspoon cornstarch

1 cup cooked chicken, chopped

2 tablespoons celery, chopped

1 tablespoon green onions, chopped

1 tablespoon almonds, finely chopped

1 cup rice, cooked

1 cup lettuce, shredded

● Combine crushed pineapple, vinegar, and cornstarch in a small saucepan. Stir to dissolve cornstarch. Cook mixture over medium heat until clear and thickened. Cool completely. Combine chicken, celery, green onions, and almonds in a bowl. Add pineapple mixture. Toss to mix. Serve sweet and sour chicken over rice; then top with shredded lettuce.

EACH SERVING: ABOUT 230 CALORIES, 26 G PROTEIN, 18 G CARBOHYDRATE,
6 G TOTAL FAT (1 G SATURATED), 60 MG CHOLESTEROL, 211 MG SODIUM.
EXCHANGE, 1 SERVING: 2 1/2 LEAN MEAT, 1/2 FRUIT, 1 STARCH/BREAD

Sweet and Sour Chicken with Rice

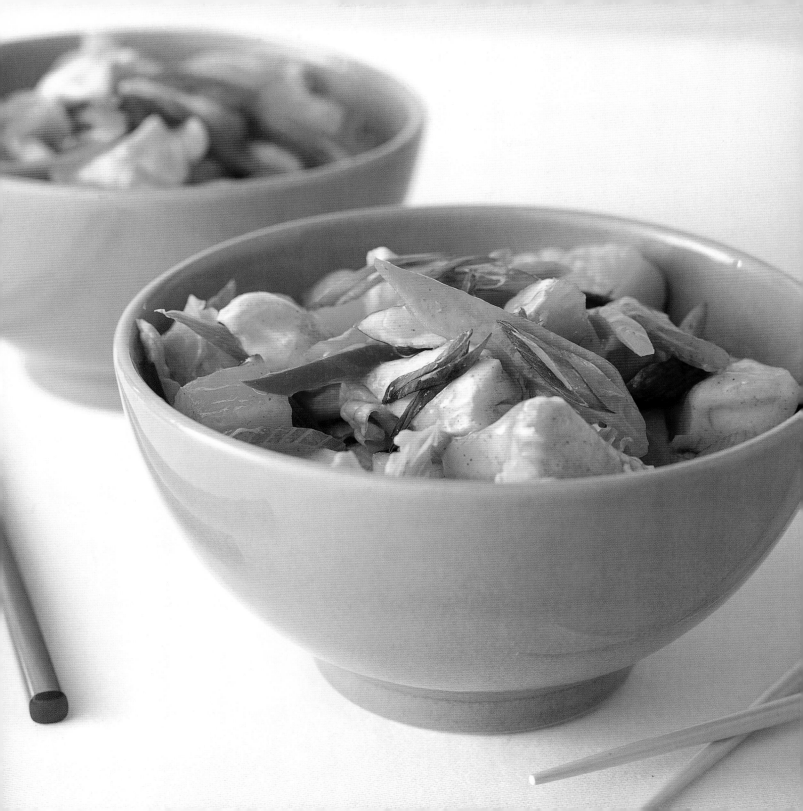

PREP TIME: 15 MINUTES   COOK TIME: 12 TO 15 MINUTES

Chicken Breast Parmesan

MAKES 2 SERVINGS

1 4-ounce chicken breast, boned
2 tablespoons all-purpose flour
dash salt
dash pepper
dash oregano
1/2 teaspoon olive oil
1 tablespoon grated Parmesan cheese

● Remove skin from chicken breast. Place the chicken breast between two pieces of plastic wrap or waxed paper. Using the bottom of a plate, rolling pin, or mallet, flatten chicken breast slightly. Combine flour, salt, pepper, and oregano in a bowl. Stir to mix. Pat flour mixture on both sides of the chicken breast. Heat oil in a nonstick skillet. Add chicken breast and brown both sides. Place chicken breast on hot ovenproof plate or platter. Sprinkle cheese over top of chicken breast. Bake chicken breast in a preheated 400°F oven for 12 to 15 minutes.

EACH SERVING: ABOUT 113 CALORIES, 15G PROTEIN, 6 G CARBOHYDRATE,
3 G TOTAL FAT (1 G SATURATED), 35 MG CHOLESTEROL, 161 MG SODIUM.
EXCHANGE, 1 SERVING: 2 LEAN MEAT

PREP TIME: 10 MINUTES

Turkey and Water-Chestnut Wraps

MAKES 2 SERVINGS

1 cup cooked turkey, chopped
2 tablespoons celery, finely chopped
2 tablespoons water chestnuts, finely chopped
1/4 cup low-calorie salad dressing
1/2 teaspoon poultry seasoning
salt and pepper to taste
2 small flour tortillas

● Combine turkey, celery, water chestnuts, salad dressing, poultry seasoning, salt, and pepper in a bowl. Toss to mix. Spread half the mixture on each tortilla and roll up.

EACH SERVING: ABOUT 317 CALORIES, 25 G PROTEIN, 31 G CARBOHYDRATE,
10 G TOTAL FAT (2 G SATURATED), 58 MG CHOLESTEROL, 890 MG SODIUM.
EXCHANGE, 1 SERVING: 2 STARCH/BREAD, 3 LEAN MEAT

Turkey and Water-Chestnut Wraps

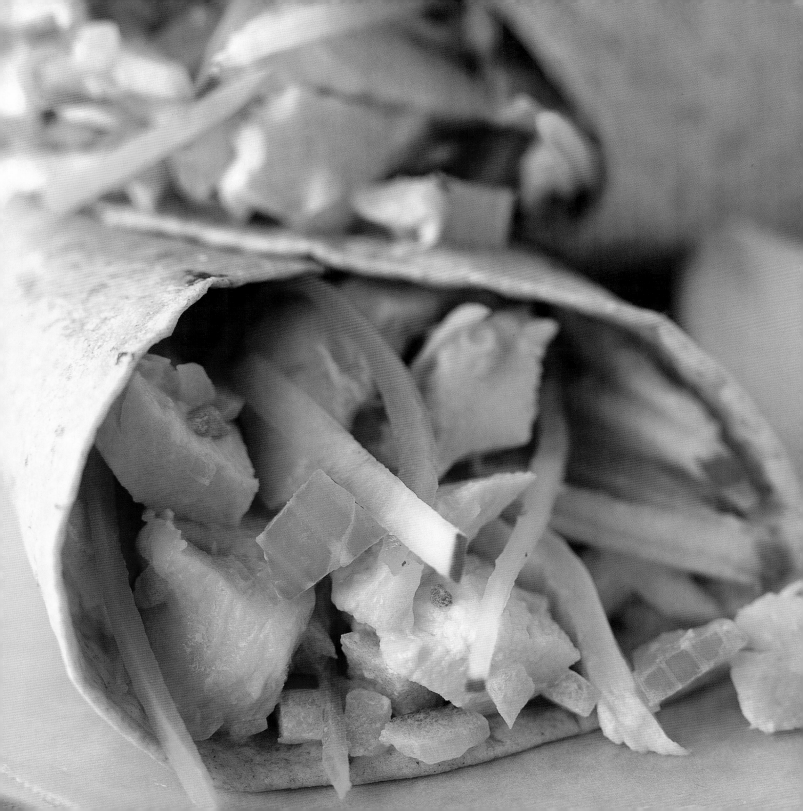

Crowned Chicken Breasts

MAKES 4 SERVINGS

This is one of my daughter Beth Ann's favorite entrées.

3 *tablespoons margarine*
4 *4-ounce chicken breasts, boned*
2 *tablespoons celery, very finely chopped*
1 *tablespoon onion, very finely chopped*
2 *cups mushrooms*
2 *tablespoons flour*

• Melt 1 tablespoon of the margarine in a nonstick skillet. Curl or roll up breasts and fasten with toothpicks or poultry pins. Over low heat, brown chicken breasts on all sides. Lift and place breasts, skin side up, in a 10-inch pie pan. Remove toothpicks or pins. In the same skillet, melt 1 tablespoon of the margarine. Add celery and onion; cook and stir until onion is tender. Slice mushrooms in half (if mushrooms are large, slice into thirds). Add mushrooms to pan and continue cooking; occasionally flip with a spatula until mushrooms are partially tender. Remove celery, onion, and mushrooms from pan and set aside. Melt remaining 1 tablespoon margarine in the skillet and stir in the flour. Cook and stir until flour is brown. Add enough water to make a thin sauce. Return mushrooms, onions, and celery to skillet and stir to mix. Pour mushroom sauce over chicken breasts. Cover with aluminum foil. Bake at 300°F for 40 to 45 minutes.

EACH SERVING: ABOUT 374 CALORIES, 56 G PROTEIN, 5 G CARBOHYDRATE, 13 G TOTAL FAT (2 G SATURATED), 137 MG CHOLESTEROL, 158 MG SODIUM. EXCHANGE, 1 SERVING: 2 HIGH-FAT MEAT

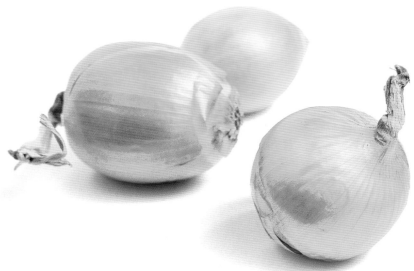

PREP TIME: 10 MINUTES   COOK TIME: 20 MINUTES
(REFRIGERATE OVERNIGHT)

Chicken with Ginger

MAKES 2 SERVINGS

2 chicken thighs

1/4 cup cider vinegar

3 tablespoons Worcestershire sauce

1/4 teaspoon ground ginger

● Clean chicken thighs and then remove skin. Combine remaining ingredients in a bowl. Stir to blend. Place thighs in marinade. Cover and refrigerate at least 8 hours or overnight. Place chicken thighs over medium-hot coals on barbecue grill or under oven broiler on middle rack. Turn and baste with marinade every 5 minutes for 15 to 20 minutes. Test for doneness by inserting a fork into the chicken; the meat should move easily.

EACH SERVING: ABOUT 98 CALORIES, 14 G PROTEIN, 4 G CARBOHYDRATE,
3 G TOTAL FAT (1 G SATURATED), 57 MG CHOLESTEROL, 1,606 MG SODIUM.
EXCHANGE: 1 LEAN MEAT

PREP TIME: 15 MINUTES   COOK TIME: 45 MINUTES

Paprika and Onion Chicken

MAKES 2 SERVINGS

1/2 white onion, chopped

1 tablespoon low-calorie margarine

2 chicken thighs

2 teaspoons paprika

1 stalk celery, chopped

1 tomato, chopped

salt and pepper to taste

● Sauté the onion in the margarine until translucent. Add the chicken thighs and brown on both sides. Remove chicken thighs. Add remaining ingredients and small amount of water. Stir to blend. Replace chicken thighs in pan. Cover and simmer for 20 to 35 minutes or until chicken is tender; add small amount of extra water, if needed.

EACH SERVING: ABOUT 257 CALORIES, 18 G PROTEIN, 7 G CARBOHYDRATE,
18 G TOTAL FAT (5 G SATURATED), 79 MG CHOLESTEROL, 166 MG SODIUM.
EXCHANGE, EACH SERVING: 2 MEDIUM-FAT MEAT

Chicken Livers and Herbs

MAKES 2 SERVINGS

1 tablespoon low-calorie margarine

2 tablespoons red onion, chopped

1/2 cup cleaned chicken livers

1 teaspoon sage

1/2 teaspoon oregano

1/8 teaspoon fennel seed, crushed

salt and pepper to taste

● Melt the margarine in a skillet. Sauté onion until slightly brown. Add chicken livers, herbs, fennel, salt, and pepper. Sauté over high heat until the pink liver juices disappear. Do not overcook. Slide out onto heated plate or heated bed of wilted lettuce.

EACH SERVING: ABOUT 111 CALORIES, 12 G PROTEIN, 4 G CARBOHYDRATE, 5 G TOTAL FAT (1 G SATURATED), 281 MG CHOLESTEROL, 121 MG SODIUM. EXCHANGE, EACH SERVING: 1 MEDIUM-FAT MEAT

Chicken Sauté

MAKES 2 SERVINGS

4 ounces skinned and boned chicken breast

3 tablespoons whole-wheat flour

1/8 teaspoon each rosemary, thyme, lemon basil

salt and pepper to taste

2 tablespoons butter

● Place the chicken breast between two pieces of plastic wrap or waxed paper. Using the bottom of a plate, rolling pin, or mallet, flatten the chicken breast to 1/4 inch. Combine remaining ingredients, except butter, in a bowl or on a piece of waxed paper. Stir to mix. Dredge the flattened chicken breast in the mixture. Melt the butter in a skillet. Then sauté the chicken breast for 2 to 3 minutes on each side.

EACH SERVING: ABOUT 203 CALORIES, 15 G PROTEIN, 8 G CARBOHYDRATE, 12 G TOTAL FAT (7 G SATURATED), 64 MG CHOLESTEROL, 155 MG SODIUM. EXCHANGE, EACH SERVING: 2 MEDIUM-FAT MEAT, 1/3 STARCH/BREAD

PREP TIME: 30 MINUTES   COOK TIME: 10 MINUTES

Eric's Chicken Wings

MAKES 1 SERVING

When I was writing the *Diabetic Gourmet Cookbook*, my son, Eric, developed this recipe. It's marvelous as either a snack or an appetizer.

3 chicken wings

1 tablespoon vegetable oil

2 tablespoons brandy

2 tablespoons water

1 tablespoon soy sauce

1 teaspoon peanut butter

1 tablespoon boiling water

1/2 teaspoon Worcestershire sauce

● First clean the chicken wings; then cut them at the joints. Discard wing ends. In a small skillet, brown the wings in the vegetable oil. Add the brandy, 1 tablespoon of the water, and the soy sauce, adding another tablespoon of the water if needed. Cover and cook over medium heat for 15 minutes. Combine the peanut butter and the boiling water in a small bowl. Stir to dissolve peanut butter; then add Worcestershire sauce. Pour over chicken wings. Cover and continue cooking for 7 to 10 minutes.

ABOUT 211 CALORIES, 11 G PROTEIN, 3 G CARBOHYDRATE, 15 G TOTAL FAT (3 G SATURATED), 38 MG CHOLESTEROL, 1,267 MG SODIUM. EXCHANGE, EACH SERVING: 1 MEDIUM-FAT MEAT

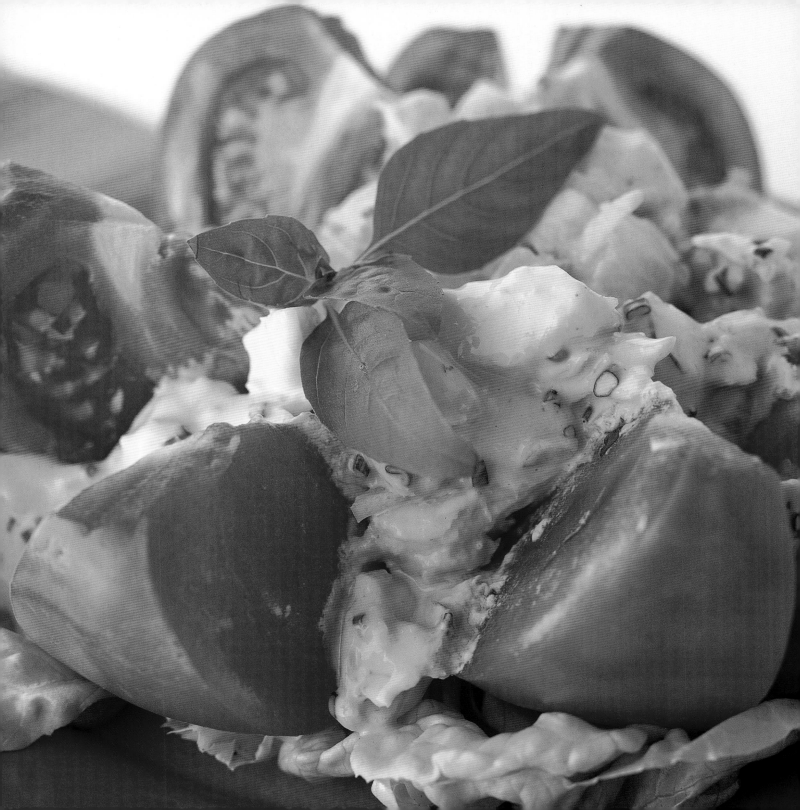

Fish & Seafood

Louis's Seafood Surprise • • Tuna Casserole

Tuna Patties • • Shrimp Egg Rolls

Salmon Salad • • White Sauce

Scalloped Crab • • Fish Florentine

Mustard Halibut Steaks • • Shrimp Delight

Great Crab • • Shrimp Soufflé

Marinated Crab Legs • • Shrimp Bouillabaisse

Teriyaki Marinade • • Tomato Stuffed with Crab Louis

Oysters on the Shell • • Venetian Seafood

Long Island Boil • • Sautéed Salmon

French Toasted Salmon Sandwiches • • Scallop Bake

Baked Turbot • • Shrimp Creole

Swordfish Amandine • • Creole Sauce

Fried Oysters • • Salmon Patties

Seafood Medley • • Shrimp Filling (for sandwiches)

Shrimp and Broccoli Chinese Style • • Crab Filling (for sandwiches)

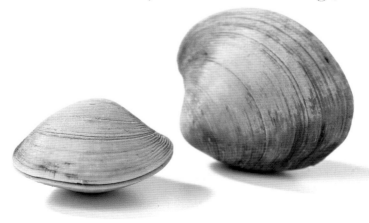

PREP TIME: 15 MINUTES   COOK TIME: 45 MINUTES

Louis's Seafood Surprise

MAKES 8 SERVINGS

3 tomatoes

1/3 cup fresh green beans

1/2 can tomato soup

3 cups water

1 cup celery, chopped

1 cup carrots, grated

1 cup mushrooms, sliced

1/2 cup cabbage, shredded

1/2 cup onion, chopped

1/4 cup corn

1/4 cup peas

1 clove garlic, finely chopped

2 teaspoons salt

1/2 teaspoon dried basil

1/2 teaspoon parsley flakes

1/4 teaspoon dried sweet marjoram

1/4 teaspoon ground red pepper

8 ounces sole, cut into bite-size pieces

4 ounces small shrimp

4 ounces crabmeat, cut into bite-size pieces

● Core but do not peel tomatoes; cut into medium-size pieces. Clean and trim beans. Combine tomato soup, water, and all vegetables and garlic in large saucepan. Add salt, basil, parsley flakes, sweet marjoram, and red pepper. Cover tightly and cook over low heat until tomatoes are soft. Add sole, shrimp, and crab. Cook until sole is firm but not broken. Serve in heated soup bowls.

EACH SERVING: ABOUT 98 CALORIES, 13 G PROTEIN, 10 G CARBOHYDRATE, 1 G TOTAL FAT (TRACE SATURATED), 41 MG CHOLESTEROL, 887 MG SODIUM. EXCHANGE, 1 SERVING: 1/2 BREAD, 1 MEDIUM-FAT MEAT

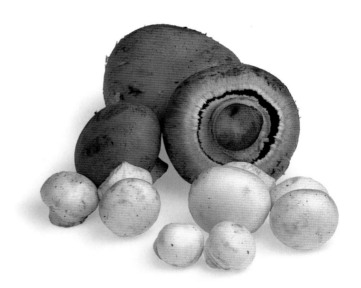

Tuna Patties

PREP TIME: 15 MINUTES   COOK TIME: 25 MINUTES

MAKES 6 SERVINGS

2 eggs

2 6¹/2-ounce cans chunk-light tuna in water

¹/3 cup milk

dash pepper

1 teaspoon lemon juice

2 tablespoons pickle relish

1 cup bran flakes cereal

fresh parsley, chopped

● Beat eggs lightly. Add remaining ingredients except parsley. Mix well. Shape into 6 patties. Place on lightly greased baking sheet. Bake at 350°F about 25 minutes, turning patties after 15 minutes. Sprinkle with parsley.

EACH SERVING: ABOUT 129 CALORIES, 19 G PROTEIN, 8 G CARBOHYDRATE, 2 G TOTAL FAT (1 G SATURATED) 90 MG CHOLESTEROL, 326 MG SODIUM. EXCHANGE, 1 SERVING: 2 LEAN MEAT, 1/3 BREAD

Salmon Salad

PREP TIME: 20 MINUTES   COOK TIME: 1 MINUTE

MAKES 8 SANDWICH SERVINGS OR 16 APPETIZERS

1 8-ounce can salmon

¹/4 cup chopped onion

¹/4 cup peeled, seeded, and chopped cucumber

2 tablespoons chopped parsley

¹/2 teaspoon celery seed

2 tablespoons low-calorie salad dressing

1 tablespoon prepared mustard

1 tablespoon ketchup

8 slices bread

8 slices tomato

● Remove skin and bones from salmon. Drain thoroughly and flake. Add onion, cucumber, parsley, celery seed, salad dressing, mustard, and ketchup. Stir to mix. Spread salmon mixture on bread. Top each sandwich half with a tomato slice. Serve cold or put sandwiches on cookie sheet and place under broiler for 30 seconds. For appetizers, cut each sandwich diagonally in half.

EACH SANDWICH SERVING: ABOUT 129 CALORIES, 9 G PROTEIN, 16 G CARBOHYDRATE, 4 G TOTAL FAT (1 G SATURATED), 17 MG CHOLESTEROL, 394 MG SODIUM. EXCHANGE, 1 SANDWICH SERVING: 1 STARCH/BREAD, 3/4 LEAN MEAT EXCHANGE, 1 APPETIZER: 1/2 STARCH/BREAD, 1/2 LEAN MEAT

PREP TIME: 10 MINUTES   COOK TIME: 15 TO 20 MINUTES

Scalloped Crab

MAKES 2 SERVINGS

1 cup crabmeat

1/2 cup soda-cracker crumbs

2 teaspoons low-calorie margarine

1/3 cup skim milk

salt and pepper to taste

● Arrange a layer of crab on the bottom of a baking dish sprayed with vegetable oil. Sprinkle cracker crumbs over the top. Dot with the margarine. Pour in milk and then sprinkle with salt and pepper. Bake at 375°F for 15 to 20 minutes or until milk is completely absorbed.

EACH SERVING: ABOUT 221 CALORIES, 24 G PROTEIN, 15 G CARBOHYDRATE, 7 G TOTAL FAT (2 G SATURATED), 53 MG CHOLESTEROL, 1,242 MG SODIUM. EXCHANGE, 1 SERVING: 1¹/2 STARCH/BREAD, 1 MEDIUM-FAT MEAT

PREP TIME: 10 MINUTES   COOK TIME: 5 MINUTES

Mustard Halibut Steaks

MAKES 1 SERVING

3-ounce halibut steak

1 teaspoon margarine

1 teaspoon lemon juice

1/2 teaspoon Dijon mustard

dash grated lemon rind

dash sugar replacement

salt to taste

● Wash and dry halibut thoroughly. Melt margarine; brush on both sides of halibut. Lay on broiler pan. Brush top with mixture of lemon juice, Dijon mustard, and seasonings. Broil 5 to 6 inches from heat for 3 to 4 minutes. Turn halibut; repeat on second side.

ABOUT 136 CALORIES, 18 G PROTEIN, 1 G CARBOHYDRATE, 7 G TOTAL FAT (1 G SATURATED), 27 MG CHOLESTEROL, 75 MG SODIUM. EXCHANGE: 1 LEAN MEAT, 1 FAT

Mustard Halibut Steaks

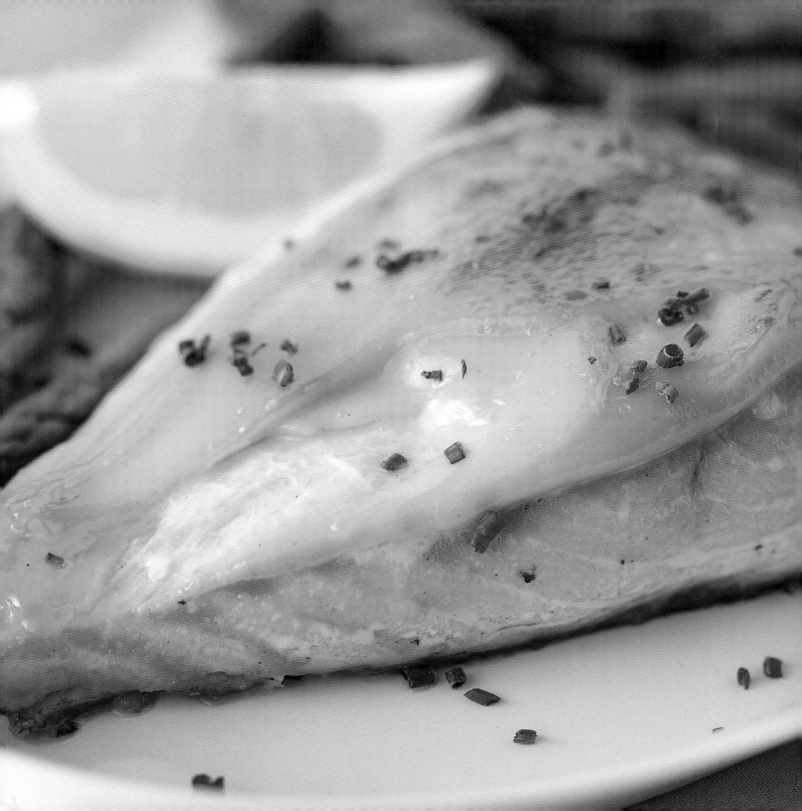

PREP TIME: 5 MINUTES   COOK TIME: 10 MINUTES

Great Crab

MAKES 1 SERVING

1 teaspoon butter

dash lemon juice

dash parsley

dash rosemary

dash salt

dash paprika

2 ounces crabmeat

● Melt butter in small saucepan. Mix in lemon juice and seasonings. Add crabmeat. Toss to coat and heat.

ABOUT 83 CALORIES, 11 G PROTEIN, 0 G CARBOHYDRATE,
4 G TOTAL FAT (1 G SATURATED), 30 MG CHOLESTEROL, 317 MG SODIUM.
EXCHANGE: 2 LEAN MEAT, 1 FAT

PREP TIME: 5 MINUTES   (MARINATE 2 TO 3 HOURS)

Marinated Crab Legs

MAKES 16 SERVINGS

1/2 cup Teriyaki Marinade (page opposite)

1/3 cup lemon juice

1/2 cup water

1 teaspoon dried basil

1 to 2 pounds cooked crab legs, shelled

● Combine marinade, lemon juice, water, and basil. Add crab legs. (If necessary, add more water to cover legs.) Marinate 2 to 3 hours.

EACH SERVING: ABOUT 29 CALORIES, 5 G PROTEIN, 1 G CARBOHYDRATE,
TRACE TOTAL FAT (0 G SATURATED), 12 MG CHOLESTEROL, 870 MG SODIUM.
EXCHANGE, 1 OUNCE: 1 LEAN MEAT

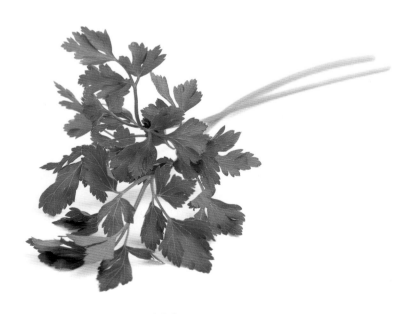

Teriyaki Marinade

MAKES 2/3 CUP

1/3 cup soy sauce

2 tablespoons wine vinegar

2 tablespoons sugar replacement

2 teaspoons salt

1 teaspoon ginger, powdered

1/2 teaspoon garlic powder

● Blend all ingredients well.

CALORIES: NEGLIGIBLE, EXCHANGE: NEGLIGIBLE

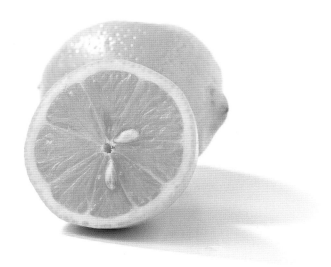

Oysters on the Shell

MAKES 1 SERVING

2 ounces oysters

2 tablespoons mushroom pieces

1 teaspoon onion, diced

1/4 cup vegetable broth

1 slice bread, finely crumbled

1/4 teaspoon lemon juice

salt and pepper to taste

1 oyster shell

1/4 ounce Cheddar cheese, grated

● Cook oysters in small amount of boiling salted water until edges start to curl. Drain (reserve some liquid). Combine mushrooms, onion, and broth in saucepan. Bring to a boil. Reduce heat. Add bread crumbs; stir to mix. Remove from heat. Add lemon juice and enough reserved oyster liquid to moisten bread-crumb mixture thoroughly. Add oysters, salt, and pepper. Heap into shell or small baking dish. Top with cheese. Broil until cheese melts.

**ABOUT 164 CALORIES, 14 G PROTEIN, 18 G CARBOHYDRATE,
4 G TOTAL FAT (2 G SATURATED), 20 MG CHOLESTEROL, 613 MG SODIUM.
EXCHANGE: 2 1/2 LEAN MEAT, 1 BREAD**

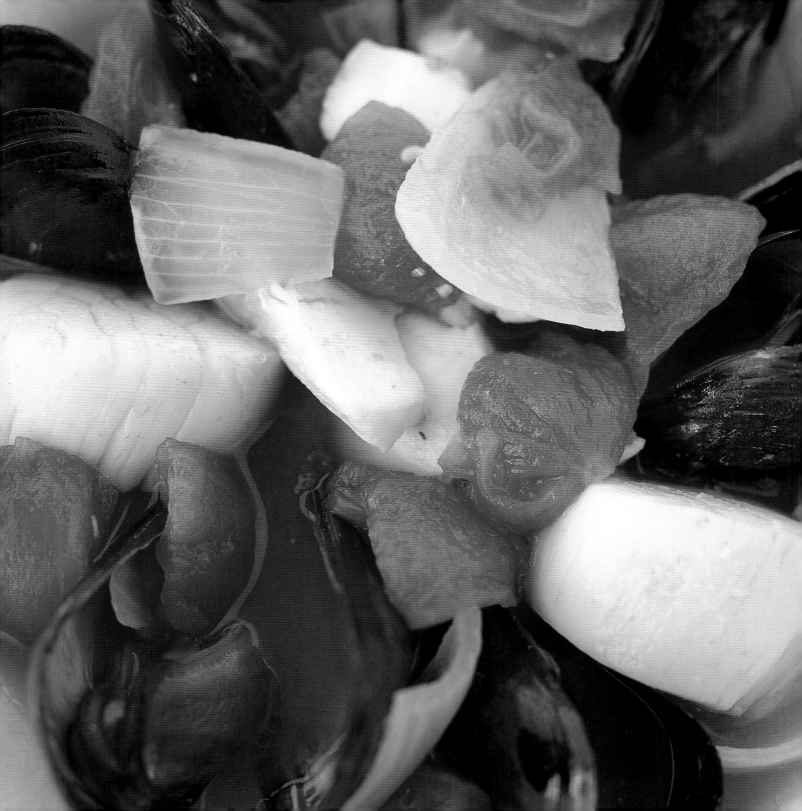

PREP TIME: 10 MINUTES   COOK TIME: 45 MINUTES
(SOAK OVERNIGHT)

Long Island Boil

MAKES 1 SERVING

1 ounce mussels

1 tomato, peeled and quartered

1 onion, cut into large chunks

1/2 teaspoon garlic powder

1 teaspoon parsley

1 ounce halibut, cut into chunks

1 ounce scallops

salt and pepper to taste

● Wash mussels thoroughly. Soak in cold water overnight. Steam mussels until shells open; remove mussels from shells. Combine tomato, onion, garlic powder, and parsley. Simmer for 15 minutes. Add halibut and scallops. Cover; simmer 10 minutes. Add mussels, salt, and pepper. Heat thoroughly.

**ABOUT 145 CALORIES, 17 G PROTEIN, 16 G CARBOHYDRATE,
2 G TOTAL FAT (TRACE SATURATED), 26 MG CHOLESTEROL, 193 MG SODIUM.
EXCHANGE: 3 LEAN MEAT, 1 VEGETABLE**

PREP TIME: 20 MINUTES   COOK TIME: 15 MINUTES

French Toasted Salmon Sandwiches

MAKES 8 SERVINGS

1 8-ounce can salmon

3 tablespoons low-calorie salad dressing

2 teaspoons grated onion

1/2 teaspoon salt

1/8 teaspoon black pepper

8 slices low-calorie white bread

1 egg

1 tablespoon skim milk

● Drain salmon, reserving liquid. Remove skin and bones, and flake. Add salad dressing, onion, salt, and pepper to salmon; then toss to mix. Spread salmon mixture on 4 slices of bread; then top each with remaining slices of bread. Combine egg, skim milk, and reserved salmon liquid in a flat bowl. With a whip or fork, beat to blend. Dip sandwiches into the egg mixture, coating both sides. Fry in a skillet sprayed with vegetable oil over medium heat until browned on both sides. Cut in half. Serve hot.

**EACH SERVING: ABOUT 130 CALORIES, 9 G PROTEIN, 14 G CARBOHYDRATE,
4 G TOTAL FAT (1 G SATURATED), 44 MG CHOLESTEROL, 366 MG SODIUM.
EXCHANGE, 1 SERVING: 1 LEAN MEAT, 1/2 STARCH/BREAD**

Long Island Boil

Baked Turbot

MAKES 2 SERVINGS

8 ounces turbot fillet

2 teaspoons margarine

2 teaspoons lemon juice

dash each salt, pepper, paprika, and parsley

● Clean turbot fillet thoroughly; pat dry. Melt margarine; brush on both sides of fillet. Place on aluminum foil. Sprinkle with lemon juice, then seasonings. Wrap up fillet securely; lay in cake pan. Bake at 350°F for 30 to 40 minutes. Slide fish from foil onto warm serving plate.

EACH SERVING: ABOUT 143 CALORIES, 18 G PROTEIN, 1 G CARBOHYDRATE, 7 G TOTAL FAT (2 G SATURATED), 54 MG CHOLESTEROL, 221 MG SODIUM. EXCHANGE, EACH SERVING: 4 MEDIUM-FAT MEAT, 1 FAT

Swordfish Amandine

MAKES 1 SERVING

2 tablespoons chopped almonds

4 ounces swordfish steak

1 teaspoon chopped parsley

1 teaspoon lemon juice

1 tablespoon dry sherry

● Brown almonds in a skillet sprayed with vegetable oil. Set aside. Place swordfish in a metal pie pan. Spray fish with vegetable oil. Combine parsley, lemon juice, and sherry in a small bowl. Spoon half the sauce over the fish. Broil for 10 minutes, basting lightly after 5 minutes. Turn fish and then coat with vegetable-oil spray again. Spoon half the remaining sauce over fish. Replace in broiler and cook for 10 minutes more, basting after 5 minutes. Place on warmed plate, and garnish with almonds.

ABOUT 263 CALORIES, 27 G PROTEIN, 5 G CARBOHYDRATE, 14 G TOTAL FAT (2 G SATURATED), 44 MG CHOLESTEROL, 109 MG SODIUM. EXCHANGE: 2 HIGH-FAT MEAT

Fried Oysters

MAKES 1 SERVING

1 tablespoon all-purpose flour

2 tablespoons soda-cracker crumbs, very fine

6 oysters

1 tablespoon low-calorie margarine

● Combine flour and cracker crumbs in a small bowl. Roll oysters in crumb-flour mixture. Melt margarine in small skillet. Then sauté oysters until golden brown.

ABOUT 292 CALORIES, 11 G PROTEIN, 22 G CARBOHYDRATE, 18 G TOTAL FAT
(2 G SATURATED), 43 MG CHOLESTEROL, 421 MG SODIUM.
EXCHANGE: 1 MEDIUM-FAT MEAT, 1 STARCH/BREAD, 1 FAT

Seafood Medley

MAKES 1 SERVING

1 ounce chunk tuna

1 ounce small shrimp, cooked

1 teaspoon lemon juice

1/2 egg, hard-boiled and chopped

1 teaspoon green onion, sliced

1 lettuce leaf

● Combine all ingredients, except lettuce. Chill thoroughly before serving on lettuce leaf with favorite dressing.

ABOUT 102 CALORIES, 16 G PROTEIN, 1 G CARBOHYDRATE,
3 G TOTAL FAT (1 G SATURATED), 170 MG CHOLESTEROL, 191 MG SODIUM.
EXCHANGE: 2 1/2 MEDIUM-FAT MEAT, 1/4 VEGETABLE

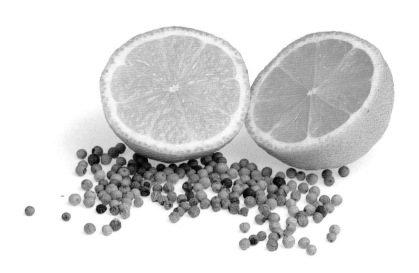

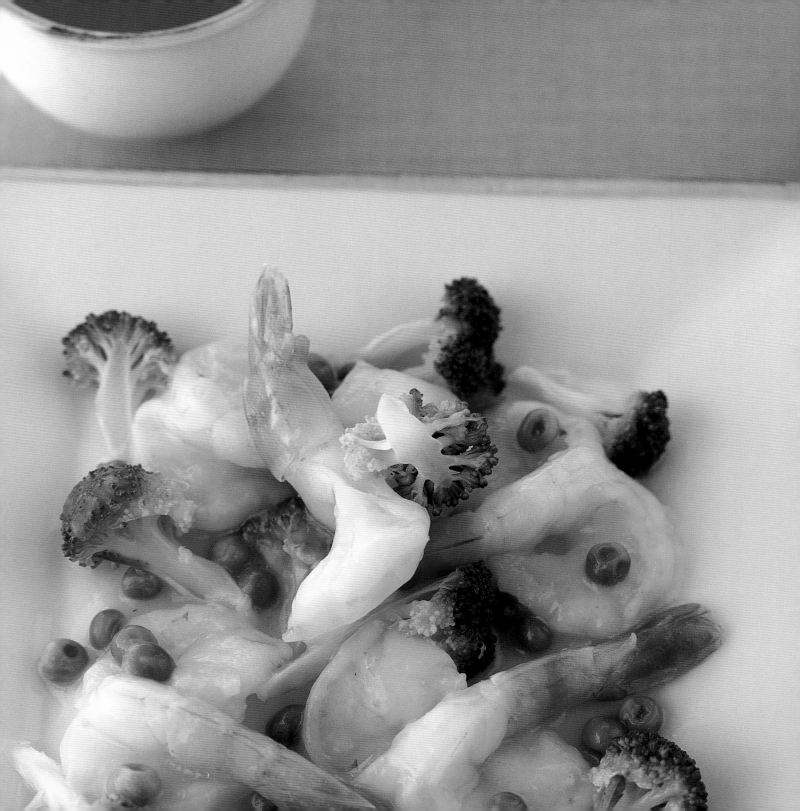

Shrimp and Broccoli Chinese Style

MAKES 4 SERVINGS

Make sure you do not overcook this dish. Chinese food should be crispy.

10 ounces shrimp, cleaned
1/4 cup vegetable oil
1 clove garlic, minced
2 cups broccoli florets
2/3 cup and 2 tablespoons water
1 teaspoon salt
2 cups fresh or frozen peas
1 tablespoon cornstarch

● Cut shrimp into 1/2-inch lengths. Heat oil in wok or skillet, add garlic, and cook until transparent. Stir in the shrimp and cook just until their color changes. Remove shrimp from wok and keep hot. Add broccoli to wok and cook 1 minute. Carefully add 2/3 cup water and salt; cover and bring water to the boiling point. Add peas, cook 5 minutes. Return shrimp to wok. Blend cornstarch with 2 tablespoons cold water; add to pan. Simmer and stir until mixture thickens and is clear.

EACH SERVING: ABOUT 276 CALORIES, 19 G PROTEIN, 15 G CARBOHYDRATE, 16 G TOTAL FAT (1 G SATURATED), 108 MG CHOLESTEROL, 697 MG SODIUM. EXCHANGE, 1 SERVING: 1/2 BREAD, 1 VEGETABLE, 2 MEDIUM-FAT MEAT

Tuna Casserole

MAKES 6 SERVINGS

1 7-ounce can tuna in water
1 10-ounce can cream of mushroom soup
2 cups crushed potato chips
2 tablespoons minced chives

● Combine all ingredients in a bowl. Toss to mix. Turn into a casserole or baking dish, sprayed with vegetable oil. Bake at 375°F for 30 to 35 minutes.

EACH SERVING: ABOUT 493 CALORIES, 15 G PROTEIN, 44 G CARBOHYDRATE, 30 G TOTAL FAT (5 G SATURATED), 10 MG CHOLESTEROL, 793 MG SODIUM. EXCHANGE, 1 SERVING: 1 STARCH/BREAD, 1/2 LEAN MEAT

Shrimp and Broccoli Chinese Style

PREP TIME: 20 MINUTES   COOK TIME: 10 MINUTES

Shrimp Egg Rolls

MAKES 20 SERVINGS

FILLING

5 dried Chinese mushrooms

1/8-inch gingerroot

8 ounces shrimp

2 cloves garlic

1 leek, chopped

2 carrots, chopped

2 tablespoons olive oil

1 cup water chestnuts, sliced

2 cups bean sprouts

2 tablespoons soy sauce

1/2 teaspoon salt

1/4 teaspoon black pepper

1 tablespoon cornstarch

1 tablespoon cold water

20 egg-roll wrappers

1 egg, slightly beaten

fat for deep-frying

• Remove hard stems from mushrooms; then discard. Soak mushrooms in very hot water for about 20 minutes or until soft. Drain. Slice thin. Using steel blade of food processor, with machine running, drop gingerroot through feeder tube. Process until minced. Sprinkle over shrimp and set aside. With food processor running, drop in garlic, leek, and carrot pieces. Process until coarsely chopped. Heat the olive oil in a wok or skillet. Then add the chopped garlic, leek, and carrot, along with the sliced mushrooms, sliced water chestnuts, bean sprouts, soy sauce, salt, and pepper. Stir-fry for 30 seconds; then cover and cook for 30 more seconds. Add shrimp. Stir-fry until shrimp is pink. Combine cornstarch and cold water in a small bowl. Stir to blend. Pour into shrimp mixture. While stirring, cook lightly until mixture thickens. Remove mixture from wok and cool slightly. Place 2 tablespoons of filling in center of each egg-roll wrapper. Fold the corner of wrapper over filling; then fold in the two side corners. Brush the remaining corner with slightly beaten egg. Roll up. Place on lightly floured surface until ready to fry. Deep-fry in fat at 375°F until golden brown. Serve with Sweet Sauce.

Sweet Sauce

2 4-ounce jars apricot baby food

3 tablespoons white vinegar

3 tablespoons cold water

1 tablespoon granulated sugar replacement

2 teaspoons cornstarch

• Combine all ingredients in a saucepan. Stir to blend. While stirring, cook sauce over low heat until it thickens.

EACH SERVING: ABOUT 149 CALORIES, 7 G PROTEIN, 25 G CARBOHYDRATE, 2 G TOTAL FAT (TRACE SATURATED), 36 MG CHOLESTEROL, 380 MG SODIUM. EXCHANGE, 1 SERVING: 1/4 LEAN MEAT; 1/5 FRUIT

White Sauce

MAKES 1/2 CUP

2 tablespoons butter

1 1/2 tablespoon flour

1/4 teaspoon salt

1 teaspoon Worcestershire sauce

1 cup skim milk

Melt margarine. Add flour, salt, and Worcestershire. Blend thoroughly. Add skim milk. Cook until slightly thickened.

ABOUT 334 CALORIES, 10 G PROTEIN, 21 G CARBOHYDRATE, 23 G TOTAL FAT (4 G SATURATED), 5 MG CHOLESTEROL, 1,353 MG SODIUM. EXCHANGE, 1/2 CUP: 1 BREAD, 1/2 HIGH-FAT MEAT

Fish Florentine

MAKES 6 SERVINGS

2 tablespoons onion, chopped

1/2 cup mushrooms, chopped

1 tablespoon margarine

2 cups cooked spinach, well drained

1 teaspoon lemon juice

1 cup White Sauce (previous recipe)

3 ounces Cheddar cheese, grated

12 ounces cooked fish, flaked

● Sauté onion and mushrooms in margarine until onion is transparent. Add spinach and lemon juice; mix well. Pour into baking dish or 6 individual baking dishes coated with vegetable cooking spray. Cover with 1/2 cup of the White Sauce. Sprinkle with half the cheese. Cover with fish, then with remaining sauce. Sprinkle with remaining cheese. Bake at 350°F for 20 minutes.

● Microwave: Cook on Medium for 10 minutes; turn. Cook 5 minutes more. Hold 3 minutes.

EACH SERVING, WITHOUT SAUCE: ABOUT 113 CALORIES, 16 G PROTEIN, 2 G CARBOHYDRATE, 4 G TOTAL FAT (1 G SATURATED), 30 MG CHOLESTEROL, 317 MG SODIUM. EXCHANGE, 1 SERVING: 3 1/2 HIGH-FAT MEAT, 1 VEGETABLE, 1 BREAD, 1/2 MILK, 1 FAT

Shrimp Delight

MAKES 2 SERVINGS

1 tablespoon minced onion

1 tablespoon chopped fresh parsley

1 tablespoon minced green pepper

1/3 cup thinly sliced mushrooms

1/2 cup skim milk

2 teaspoons all-purpose flour

dash salt

dash pepper

dash nutmeg

1/2 cup cooked shrimp

2 slices toasted bread

● In a skillet sprayed with vegetable oil, sauté onion, parsley, green pepper, and mushrooms until mushrooms are tender. Combine milk and flour in a cup or shaker bottle. Stir or shake to blend. Pour over vegetables. Add dashes of salt, pepper, and nutmeg. Then add shrimp. While stirring, cook until mixture is thickened. Spoon over toast.

EACH SERVING: ABOUT 164 CALORIES, 17 G PROTEIN, 19 G CARBOHYDRATE, 2 G TOTAL FAT (1 G SATURATED), 112 MG CHOLESTEROL, 386 MG SODIUM. EXCHANGE, 1 SERVING: 1 STARCH/BREAD, 1 LEAN MEAT, 1/4 SKIM MILK

Shrimp Soufflé

MAKES 1 SERVING

2 ounces shrimp, canned

1 egg, separated

dash thyme

dash rosemary, crushed

dash salt

dash pepper

● Chop shrimp into fine pieces. Add to beaten egg yolk and seasonings. Beat egg whites until stiff. Gently stir half of egg white into shrimp mixture. Gently fold in remaining egg white. Pour into large individual soufflé dish coated with vegetable cooking spray. (Dish should be less than two-thirds full.) Bake at 375°F for 15 to 20 minutes.

ABOUT 143 CALORIES, 19 G PROTEIN, 1 G CARBOHYDRATE, 6 G TOTAL FAT (2 G SATURATED), 311 MG CHOLESTEROL, 314 MG SODIUM. EXCHANGE: 3 LEAN MEAT

PREP TIME: 15 MINUTES   COOK TIME: 35 MINUTES

Shrimp Bouillabaisse

MAKES 6 SERVINGS

1 6-ounce can tomato paste

4 cups water

2 whole cloves

2 bay leaves

2 teaspoons salt

2 cups chopped mushrooms

1/2 cup chopped onion

1 clove garlic, minced

3/4 teaspoon curry powder

1 6-ounce package frozen cooked shrimp

1/2 cup grated American cheese

1/4 cup dry sherry

1 tablespoon all-purpose flour

● Combine tomato paste, water, cloves, bay leaves, and salt in a large saucepan. Stir to blend. Bring to a boil; then reduce heat, cover, and simmer for 10 minutes. Remove cloves and bay leaves. Add mushrooms, onion, garlic, and curry powder. Simmer until vegetables are tender. Add shrimp and cheese. Stir to blend. Combine sherry and flour in a bowl or cup. Stir to blend. Pour sherry-flour mixture into soup. While stirring, cook until slightly thickened.

EACH SERVING: ABOUT 158 CALORIES, 13 G PROTEIN, 10 G CARBOHYDRATE, 7 G TOTAL FAT (4 G SATURATED), 74 MG CHOLESTEROL, 1,355 MG SODIUM. EXCHANGE, 1 SERVING: 1/2 MEDIUM-FAT MEAT, 11/2 VEGETABLES

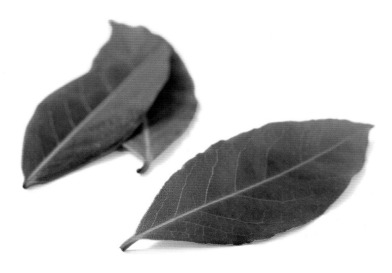

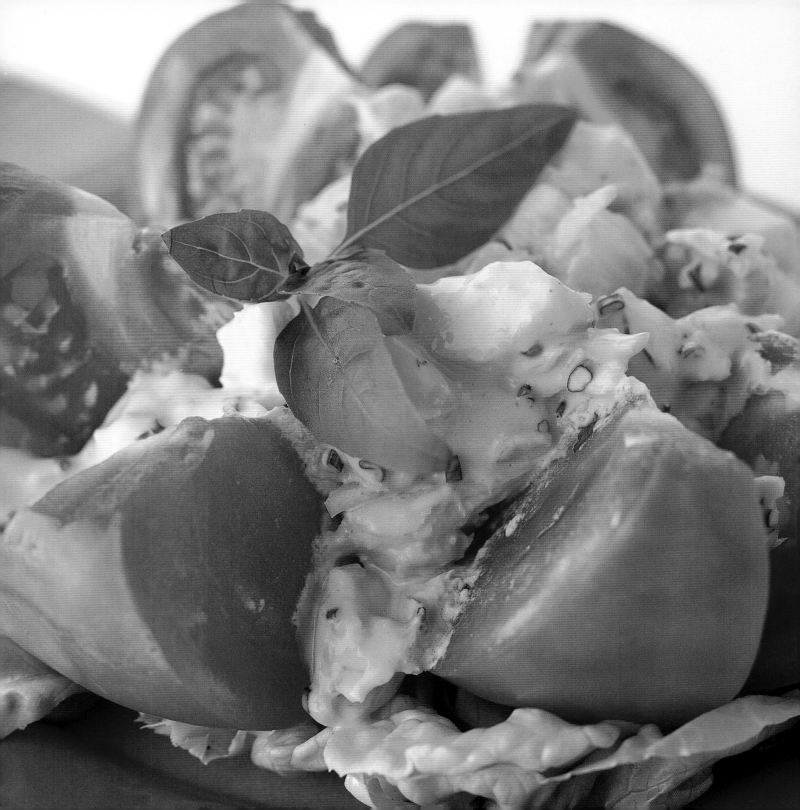

Tomato Stuffed with Crab Louis

MAKES 1 SERVING

1/2 teaspoon ketchup

1 teaspoon mayonnaise

1/4 teaspoon Worcestershire sauce

1 ounce crabmeat

1 teaspoon green onion, finely chopped

1 tablespoon celery, finely chopped

1 tablespoon green pepper, finely chopped

1 teaspoon parsley, finely chopped

3 almonds, chopped

1 tomato, peeled

1 lettuce leaf

● Blend ketchup, mayonnaise, and Worcestershire sauce; add crabmeat, green onion, celery, green pepper, parsley, and almonds. Stir to blend; chill. Cut peeled tomato into 7 sections, slicing almost to the bottom. Fill with crab mixture. Serve on lettuce leaf.

ABOUT 120 CALORIES, 9 G PROTEIN, 8 G CARBOHYDRATE, 7 G TOTAL FAT (TRACE SATURATED), 13 MG CHOLESTEROL, 444 MG SODIUM. EXCHANGE: 1 MEDIUM-FAT MEAT, 1 FAT, 1 VEGETABLE

Venetian Seafood

PREP TIME: 10 MINUTES   COOK TIME: 10 MINUTES
(MARINATE 3 TO 5 HOURS)

MAKES 1 SERVING

1/2 cup water

2 tablespoons lime juice

1 tablespoon chives, finely chopped

1 teaspoon garlic powder

1/2 teaspoon oregano

1/2 teaspoon salt

1/4 teaspoon pepper

1 ounce fresh or frozen lobster, thawed and cubed

1 ounce fresh or frozen scallops, thawed

1 ounce fresh or frozen shrimp, thawed

● Make a marinade by blending water, lime juice, and seasonings. Place thawed seafood in deep narrow dish. Pour marinade over seafood to cover. Refrigerate for 3 to 5 hours. (Stir occasionally if seafood is not completely covered with marinade.) Drain. Spray seafood with vegetable cooking spray. Place on baking sheet or dish coated with vegetable cooking spray. Broil 5 to 6 inches from heat for 5 to 6 minutes until seafood is tender. Shake baking sheet or dish occasionally to brown seafood evenly.

ABOUT 103 CALORIES, 17 G PROTEIN, 7 G CARBOHYDRATE, 1 G TOTAL FAT (TRACE SATURATED), 79 MG CHOLESTEROL, 1,331 MG SODIUM. EXCHANGE: 3 LEAN MEAT

Sautéed Salmon

PREP TIME: 5 MINUTES   COOK TIME: 15 MINUTES

MAKES 1 SERVING

1/2 onion, thinly sliced

4 ounces salmon steak, boned

1 tablespoon all-purpose flour

salt and pepper to taste

● Sauté onion in a skillet that has been sprayed with vegetable oil. When onion is evenly browned, remove and set aside. Recoat skillet with vegetable-oil spray. Flour the salmon steak on both sides; next, season with salt and pepper. Cook until fish flakes easily when tested with a fork or toothpick. Transfer to warm plate and cover with onions.

ABOUT 240 CALORIES, 26 G PROTEIN, 11 G CARBOHYDRATE, 10 G TOTAL FAT (2 G SATURATED), 70 MG CHOLESTEROL, 55 MG SODIUM. EXCHANGE: 2 MEDIUM-FAT MEAT

PREP TIME: 10 MINUTES   COOK TIME: 20 MINUTES

Scallop Bake

MAKES 10 SERVINGS

2 pounds scallops

1 cup water

1/3 cup lemon juice

2 cups mushrooms, thinly sliced

1 green pepper, diced

1/3 cup yellow onion, finely chopped

3 tablespoons all-purpose flour

1/2 teaspoon salt

1/8 teaspoon black pepper

1/2 cup diced Swiss cheese

1/4 cup grated Romano cheese

3/4 cup prepared nondairy whipped topping

paprika

● Wash and drain scallops. Bring water and lemon juice to a boil in a medium saucepan. Add scallops, mushrooms, green pepper, and onion. Reduce heat and simmer on low for 8 minutes. Remove from heat. Pour a small amount of the scallop liquid from the saucepan into a blender or small bowl. Add the flour, salt, and pepper to the liquid. Blend until smooth. Pour back into saucepan. Cook, stirring, until mixture has thickened. Stir in cheeses. While continuing to stir, cook over low heat until cheeses have melted. Remove from heat. Fold in prepared nondairy whipped topping. Divide mixture evenly among 10 lightly greased individual baking dishes. Sprinkle with paprika. Then broil until browned.

EACH SERVING: ABOUT 140 CALORIES, 19 G PROTEIN, 7 G CARBOHYDRATE, 4 G TOTAL FAT (2 G SATURATED), 40 MG CHOLESTEROL, 320 MG SODIUM. EXCHANGE, EACH SERVING: 2 LEAN MEAT, 1/2 STARCH/BREAD

Shrimp Creole

MAKES 1 SERVING

1/2 cup Creole Sauce (recipe follows)

10 small cooked shrimp

1 cup cooked rice

● Heat Creole Sauce just to a boil. Add shrimp. Remove from heat. Allow to rest 10 minutes. Serve over rice.

ABOUT 341 CALORIES, 19 G PROTEIN, 62 G CARBOHYDRATE, 2 G FAT (TRACE SATURATED), 91 MG CHOLESTEROL, 522 MG SODIUM. EXCHANGE, 2 MEAT, 2 BREAD, 1/2 VEGETABLE, 1 FAT

Creole Sauce

MAKES 4 CUPS

1 28-ounce can diced tomatoes

1 medium onion, chopped

1 green pepper

1 teaspoon paprika

1/4 teaspoon marjoram

salt and pepper to taste

● Combine all ingredients and cook over low heat for 25 minutes.

EXCHANGE: 1 VEGETABLE

Salmon Patties

MAKES 8 SERVINGS

1 16-ounce can salmon

1/4 cup dry bread crumbs

1/4 cup ketchup

1/4 cup chopped chives

1 egg

● Drain salmon thoroughly and then remove any bones or skin. Combine with remaining ingredients in a bowl. Stir to mix. Form into eight patties. Fry until browned on both sides in a skillet sprayed with vegetable oil.

EACH SERVING: ABOUT 110 CALORIES, 13 G PROTEIN, 5 G CARBOHYDRATE, 4 G TOTAL FAT (1 G SATURATED), 58 MG CHOLESTEROL, 168 MG SODIUM. EXCHANGE, EACH SERVING: 1 MEDIUM-FAT MEAT, 1/4 STARCH/BREAD

Shrimp Filling
(for sandwiches)

MAKES 4 SANDWICH FILLINGS

1 6-ounce package frozen cooked shrimp,
  thawed and drained

1/3 cup celery, finely chopped

1/3 cup bamboo shoots, finely chopped

1/4 cup bean sprouts, chopped

3 tablespoons low-calorie salad dressing

● Combine shrimp, celery, bamboo shoots, bean sprouts, and salad dressing in a bowl. (The bamboo shoots add a nutty flavor.) Toss gently to mix.

**EACH SERVING: ABOUT 68 CALORIES, 10 G PROTEIN, 2G CARBOHYDRATE,
2 G TOTAL FAT (TRACE SATURATED), 83 MG CHOLESTEROL, 191 MG SODIUM.
EXCHANGE, EACH SERVING: 1 LEAN MEAT, 1/3 FAT**

Crab Filling
(for sandwiches)

MAKES 4 SANDWICH FILLINGS

1 7-ounce can crabmeat

1/3 cup celery, finely chopped

2 tablespoons onion, finely chopped

2 tablespoons carrot, finely grated

1/3 cup low-calorie salad dressing

1 teaspoon Dijon mustard

alfalfa sprouts

● Combine crabmeat, celery, onion, carrot, salad dressing, and mustard in a bowl. Toss gently to mix. Top with alfalfa sprouts.

**EACH SERVING: ABOUT 55 CALORIES, 6 G PROTEIN, 2 G CARBOHYDRATE,
2 G TOTAL FAT (TRACE SATURATED), 14 MG CHOLESTEROL, 393 MG SODIUM.
EXCHANGE, EACH SERVING: 1/2 LEAN MEAT, 1/2 FAT**

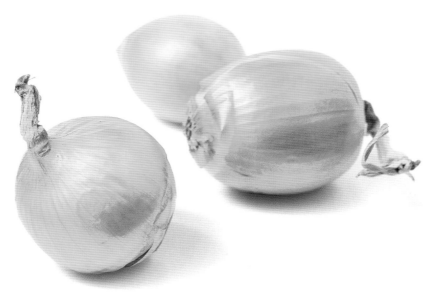

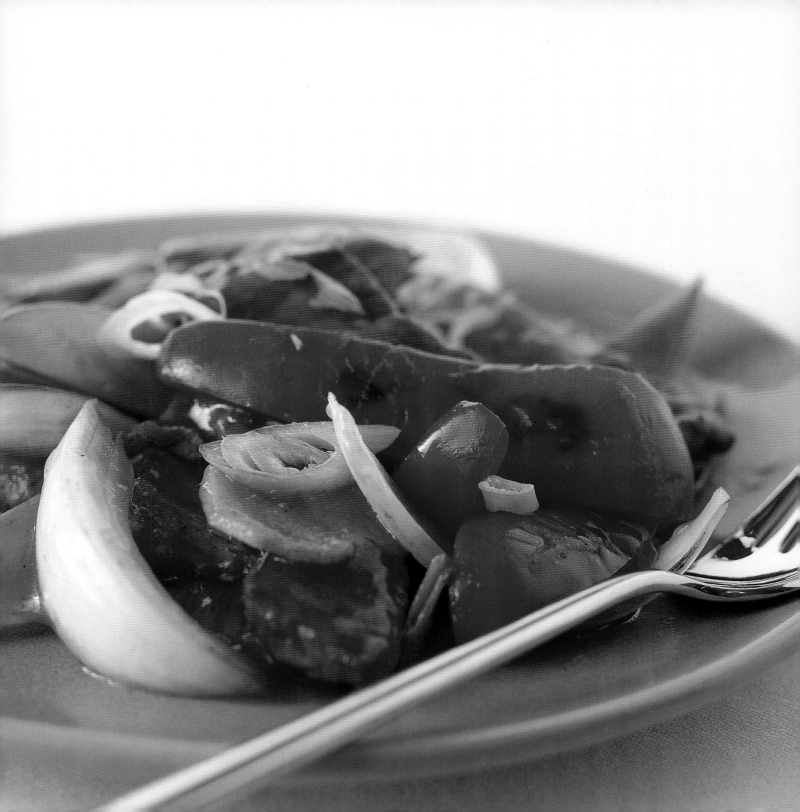

Meat

Beef Fondue •

Veal Scaloppine II •

Spicy Beef Bratwurst •

Brisket of Beef with Horseradish •

Hungarian Goulash •

Greek-Style Loukanika •

Soy Flour Meatloaf •

Peanut Pork Chops •

Mushroom-Stuffed Pork Chops •

Teriyaki Pork Steak •

Swiss Steak •

Steak Hawaiian •

Tamale Casserole •

Wheat Germ Corn Bread •

Beef with Cauliflower •

• Hot Spanish-Style Chorizo

• German Goulash

• Beef and Vegetable Stir-Fry

• Beef and Rice Casserole

• Quick Kabobs

• Beef Stroganoff

• Ham and Scalloped Potatoes

• Beef Becquee

• Dilly Beef

• Parmigiana Ham

• Sweet and Sour Pork

• Curried Meatballs

• Beef Beauties

• Pile-High Porkies

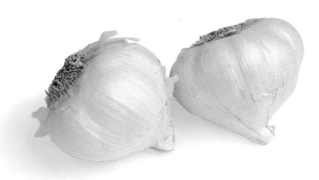

Beef Fondue

MAKES 6 SERVINGS

1 small tomato

2 cups beef broth

1 bay leaf

1/2 teaspoon rosemary, ground

6 ounces sirloin steak, cut into bite-size cubes

● Peel and crush tomato. Place beef broth, tomato, bay leaf, and rosemary in saucepan; heat to a boil. Pour into fondue pot; keep hot with a burner. Place steak cubes on spear. Cook in hot broth to desired doneness.

EACH SERVING: ABOUT 72 CALORIES, 7 G PROTEIN, 1 G CARBOHYDRATE, 5 G TOTAL FAT (2 G SATURATED), 19 MG CHOLESTEROL, 278 MG SODIUM. EXCHANGE, 1 SERVING: 1 HIGH-FAT MEAT

Veal Scaloppine II

MAKES 1 SERVING

2 ounces veal steak, boned

1/4 cup tomato, sieved

2 tablespoons green pepper, chopped

1 tablespoon mushroom pieces

1 tablespoon onions, chopped

1/4 teaspoon parsley

dash garlic powder

dash oregano

salt and pepper to taste

● Place veal on bottom of individual baking dish. Add remaining ingredients; cover. Bake at 350°F for 45 minutes, or until meat is tender.

● Microwave: Cook on High for 10 to 12 minutes. Turn and uncover last 2 minutes.

ABOUT 81 CALORIES, 12 G PROTEIN, 4 G CARBOHYDRATE, 2 G TOTAL FAT (1 G SATURATED), 45 MG CHOLESTEROL, 63 MG SODIUM. EXCHANGE: 2 LEAN MEAT, 1 VEGETABLE

PREP TIME: 25 MINUTES   COOK TIME: 10 MINUTES

Spicy Beef Bratwurst

MAKES 8 SERVINGS

1 egg

1/4 cup cold milk

1/4 teaspoon caraway seeds

1 teaspoon parsley flakes

1/4 teaspoon ground coriander

1 teaspoon ground dry lemon peel

1/4 teaspoon ground mace

1/4 teaspoon ground mustard

1 tablespoon onion powder

1/4 teaspoon paprika

3/4 teaspoon ground white pepper

1 teaspoon salt

1 tablespoon onion or leek, diced

1/4 teaspoon brown sugar

1 pound freshly ground beef

1 cup uncooked oatmeal

● Combine egg and milk in a large bowl. Crush caraway seeds and parsley flakes in mortar with pestle. Blend all seasonings, onions, and sugar into the liquid. Add beef and oatmeal and mix together to form sausage. Form 8 patties or links. Spray a skillet with nonstick cooking spray; heat over medium heat. Cook sausage 3 minutes per side or until brown.

EACH SERVING: ABOUT 272 CALORIES, 15 G PROTEIN, 21 G CARBOHYDRATE, 15 G
TOTAL FAT (5 G SATURATED), 69 MG CHOLESTEROL, 419 MG SODIUM.
EXCHANGE, 1 SERVING: 1 HIGH-FAT MEAT

PREP TIME: 10 MINUTES   COOK TIME: 3 HOURS

Brisket of Beef with Horseradish

MAKES 48 APPETIZER SERVINGS

3- to 4-pound beef brisket

Salt and pepper to taste

1 medium onion, sliced

1 bay leaf

1 tablespoon lemon juice

1/2 cup horseradish

● Place brisket in large kettle; add salt and pepper. Add onion, bay leaf, and enough water to cover brisket. Bring to a boil. Reduce heat and simmer for 2 hours. Remove brisket from water. Combine lemon juice and horseradish. Rub surface of brisket with horseradish mixture. Return brisket to kettle; cover. Cook 1 hour longer.

EACH SERVING: ABOUT 105 CALORIES, 7 G PROTEIN, 1 G CARBOHYDRATE, 8 G TOTAL FAT (3 G SATURATED), 27 MG CHOLESTEROL, 24 MG SODIUM. EXCHANGE, EACH SERVING: 1 MEDIUM-FAT MEAT

PREP TIME: 5 MINUTES   COOK TIME: 1 HOUR 15 MINUTES

Hungarian Goulash

MAKES 1 SERVING

1 tablespoon shortening or margarine

1 ounce lean beef, diced

1 ounce lean veal, diced

1 ounce beef kidney, diced

2 teaspoons onion, chopped

1 teaspoon green pepper, chopped

3 cherry tomatoes, halved

1/2 cup potato, diced

1/4 cup carrot, diced

1/4 teaspoon salt

dash paprika

dash pepper

dash marjoram

● Heat shortening or margarine in skillet; add meat. brown on all sides; drain. Place in individual casserole. Add remaining ingredients. Add enough water to cover. Cover casserole tightly; bake at 350°F for 1 hour.

● Microwave: Cook on high for 20 to 25 minutes. Stir halfway through cooking time.

ABOUT 292 CALORIES, 18 G PROTEIN, 14 G CARBOHYDRATE, 19 G TOTAL FAT (4 G SATURATED), 121 MG CHOLESTEROL, 688 MG SODIUM. EXCHANGE: 3 HIGH-FAT MEAT, 1 BREAD, 1 VEGETABLE

Hungarian Goulash

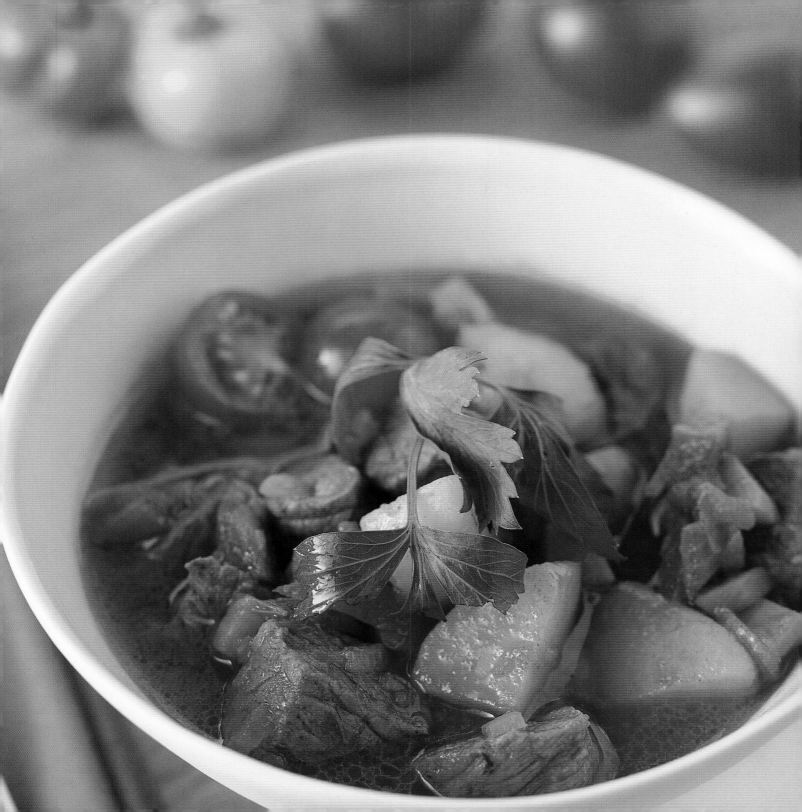

PREP TIME: 25 MINUTES   COOK TIME: 10 MINUTES

Greek-Style Loukanika

MAKES 8 PATTIES OR LINKS

Loukanika can be served as a main dish for dinner or on Greek-style bread as a luncheon meal.

1/2 cup rosé wine, chilled

2 tablespoons orange juice, chilled

1/4 teaspoon ground allspice

1/4 teaspoon ground cinnamon

1/4 teaspoon ground cumin

1 clove garlic, minced

1/4 teaspoon ground nutmeg

2 tablespoons orange peel, grated

1/4 teaspoon ground black pepper

1/2 teaspoon peppercorns, cracked

1 teaspoon salt

1 teaspoon dried savory

1/4 teaspoon brown sugar

1/2 pound freshly ground veal

1/2 pound freshly ground pork

1 cup bulgur

● Mix wine and orange juice in a large bowl. Blend all seasonings, and sugar into the liquid. Add veal, pork, and bulgur. Mix sausage with clean hands until thoroughly blended. Form 8 patties or links. Spray a skillet with nonstick cooking spray; heat over medium heat. Cook sausage 3 minutes per side or until brown.

EACH SERVING: ABOUT 192 CALORIES, 13 G PROTEIN, 15 G CARBOHYDRATE, 8 G TOTAL FT (3 G SATURATED), 43 MG CHOLESTEROL, 322 MG SODIUM. EXCHANGE, 1 SERVING: 2 MEDIUM-FAT MEAT

PREP TIME: 10 MINUTES   COOK TIME: 50 MINUTES

Soy Flour Meatloaf

MAKES 6 SERVINGS

1 pound ground meat

2 eggs

1 cup milk

2 1/2 teaspoons salt

1/2 cup soy flour

1/4 cup quick-cooking rolled oats

1/2 cup onion, minced

1/4 teaspoon black pepper

● Combine all ingredients and mix well. Shape the loaf and place in a 9" x 5" loaf pan. Bake at 350°F for 50 minutes or until done.

EACH SERVING: ABOUT 306 CALORIES, 22 G PROTEIN, 12 G CARBOHYDRATE, 19 G TOTAL FAT (7 G SATURATED), 128 MG CHOLESTEROL, 1,154MG SODIUM. EXCHANGE, 1 SERVING: 3/4 BREAD, 2 MEDIUM-FAT MEAT

PREP TIME: 10 MINUTES   COOK TIME: 15 TO 20 MINUTES

Peanut Pork Chops

MAKES 4 SERVINGS

1 egg

1/4 cup water

1/2 cup salted peanuts, finely ground

4 lean pork chops

● Beat egg with water. Place in a shallow bowl. Place ground peanuts in another shallow bowl or plastic bag. (I use the blender to grind the peanuts.) Remove and discard any excess fat from chops. Dip chops first into the egg, shaking off excess, then into the ground peanuts, covering each chop. Grill chops on a medium-high barbecue for 8 to 10 minutes on each side.

EACH SERVING: ABOUT 409 CALORIES, 31 G PROTEIN, 6 G CARBOHYDRATE, 30 G TOTAL FAT (7 G SATURATED), 128 MG CHOLESTEROL, 314 MG SODIUM. EXCHANGE, 1 SERVING: 2 HIGH-FAT MEAT

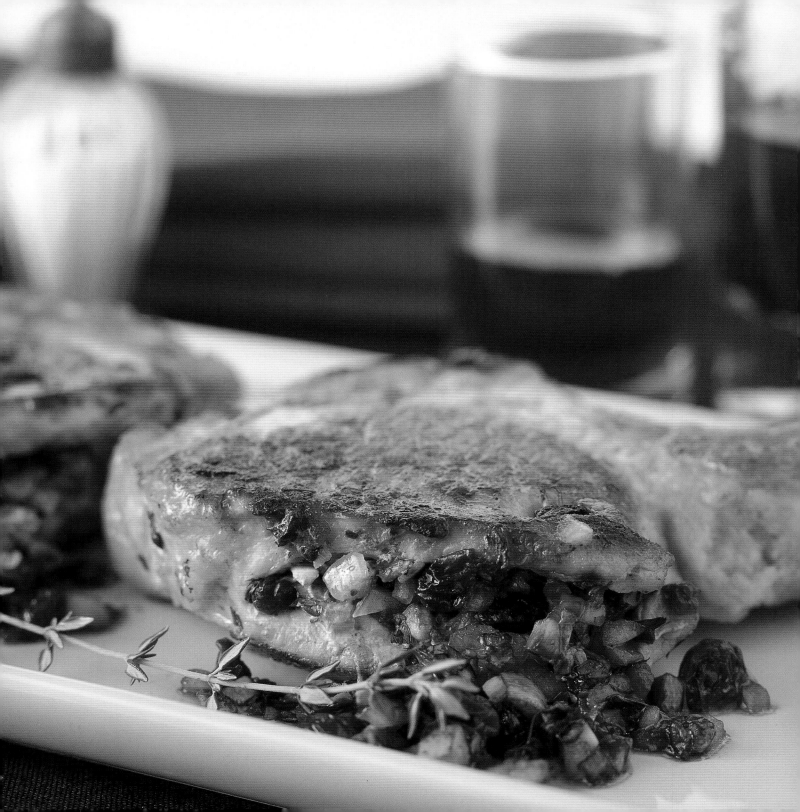

PREP TIME: 10 MINUTES   COOK TIME: 35 TO 40 MINUTES

Mushroom-Stuffed Pork Chops

MAKES 1 SERVING

2 tablespoons mushroom pieces

1 teaspoon onion, chopped

1/2 teaspoon parsley, chopped

1 teaspoon raisins, soaked

1/4 teaspoon nutmeg

1 double pork chop

● Combine ingredients for stuffing; stir to blend. Split meaty part of chop down to bone; do not split through bone. Fill with stuffing; secure with poultry pins. Place on baking sheet. Bake uncovered at 350°F for 35 to 40 minutes, or until tender. Turn once.

EABOUT 153 CALORIES, 22 G PROTEIN, 3 G CARBOHYDRATE,
5 G TOTAL FAT (2 G SATURATED), 62 MG CHOLESTEROL, 66 MG SODIUM.
EXCHANGE: 1 HIGH-FAT MEAT

PREP TIME: 10 MINUTES   COOK TIME: 5 MINUTES
(MARINATE 1 TO 2 HOURS)

Teriyaki Pork Steak

MAKES 16 2-OUNCE SERVINGS

1 pound pork steak, thinly sliced

1/2 cup soy sauce

1 tablespoon wine vinegar

2 tablespoons lemon juice

1/4 cup water

2 tablespoons sugar replacement

1 1/2 teaspoons ginger

1/2 teaspoon garlic powder

● Place slices of pork steak in shallow dish. Combine remaining ingredients; pour over pork. Marinate 1 to 2 hours; turn once. Broil pork 5 to 6 inches from heat, for 2 to 3 minutes per side. Turn and broil second side.

EACH SERVING: ABOUT 48 CALORIES, 6 G PROTEIN, 3 G CARBOHYDRATE,
1 G TOTAL FAT (TRACE SATURATED), 13 MG CHOLESTEROL, 1,734 MG SODIUM.
EXCHANGE, 1 SERVING: 1 MEDIUM-FAT MEAT

Mushroom-Stuffed Pork Chops

Swiss Steak

MAKES 1 SERVING

1 teaspoon margarine

3 ounces beef minute steak

salt and pepper to taste

1/4 cup celery, sliced

1 tablespoon onion, chopped

1/4 cup tomato, crushed

1/4 cup water

● Heat margarine until very hot. Salt and pepper the steak. Brown both sides; drain. Place in an individual baking dish. Add salt, pepper, and remaining ingredients. Cover. Bake at 375°F for 1 hour, or until steak is tender.

● Microwave: Cook on High 8 to 10 minutes. Uncover last minute.

**ABOUT 350 CALORIES, 15 G PROTEIN, 4 G CARBOHYDRATE,
30 G TOTAL FAT (12 G SATURATED), 62 MG CHOLESTEROL, 76 MG SODIUM.
EXCHANGE: 3 MEDIUM-FAT MEAT, 1 FAT**

Steak Hawaiian

MAKES 1 SERVING

3 ounces beef top round steak, sliced

1/2 teaspoon mace

2 tablespoons unsweetened pineapple juice

1 pineapple slice, unsweetened

● Pound slices of round steak with mallet or edge of plate until thin. Sprinkle both sides with mace. Place in aluminum foil. Sprinkle with pineapple juice; top with pineapple slice. Secure foil tightly. Place in baking dish. Bake at 350°F for 40 to 45 minutes.

● Microwave: Place in plastic wrap. Cook on High for 10 to 12 minutes.

**ABOUT 186 CALORIES, 19 G PROTEIN, 9 G CARBOHYDRATE,
8 G TOTAL FAT (3 G SATURATED), 52 MG CHOLESTEROL, 44 MG SODIUM.
EXCHANGE: 3 LEAN MEAT, 1 FRUIT**

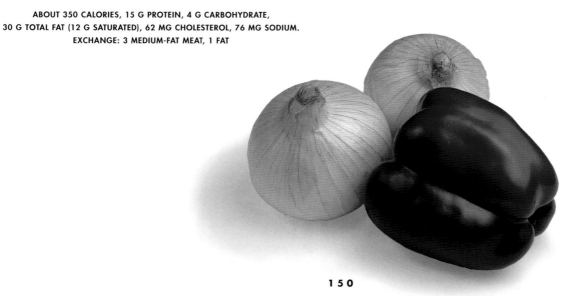

PREP TIME: 10 MINUTES   COOK TIME: 55 MINUTES

Tamale Casserole

MAKES 8 SERVINGS

1½ pounds lean ground beef

1 medium green pepper, chopped

1 large onion, chopped

1 16-ounce can whole tomatoes, undrained

1 8-ounce can tomato sauce

¼ cup wheat germ

2 teaspoons chili powder

1½ teaspoons salt

dash hot pepper sauce

1 recipe Wheat Germ Corn Bread (recipe follows)

1 cup sharp Cheddar cheese, grated

● Cook beef, green pepper, and onion over medium heat until beef is lightly browned. Drain. Stir in tomatoes, tomato sauce, wheat germ, chili powder, salt and hot pepper sauce. Simmer while preparing the batter for Wheat Germ Corn Bread. Pour hot meat mixture into greased 3-quart casserole. Spread evenly with the batter. Bake at 400°F for 25 to 30 minutes until corn bread is golden brown. Sprinkle with cheese. Bake for 2 to 3 minutes longer until cheese melts.

EACH SERVING: ABOUT 437 CALORIES, 28 G PROTEIN, 28 G CARBOHYDRATE, 24 G TOTAL FAT (9 G SATURATED), 94 MG CHOLESTEROL, 1,204 MG SODIUM. EXCHANGE: 6 MEDIUM-FAT MEAT, ½ BREAD, 1 VEGETABLE, ½ HIGH-FAT MEAT

Wheat Germ Corn Bread

MAKES 16 SERVINGS

¾ cup wheat germ

½ cup yellow cornmeal

¼ cup all-purpose flour

1½ teaspoons baking powder

½ teaspoon salt

1 egg

1 cup nonfat plain yogurt

2 tablespoons margarine, melted

● Combine wheat germ, cornmeal, flour, baking powder, and salt on waxed paper. Stir well to blend. Beat egg. Add yogurt and margarine, beating until smooth. Stir blended dry ingredients into yogurt mixture. Spread batter in greased, square 8-inch pan. Bake at 400°F for 18 to 20 minutes until wooden pick inserted in middle comes out clean.

EACH SERVING: ABOUT 69 CALORIES, 3 G PROTEIN, 9 G CARBOHYDRATE, 2 G TOTAL FAT (1 G SATURATED), 14 MG CHOLESTEROL, 81 MG SODIUM. EXCHANGE, EACH SERVING: ½ BREAD

Beef with Cauliflower

MAKES 4 SERVINGS

1/2 pound flank steak

1 teaspoon salt

1 tablespoon cornstarch

3 tablespoons soy sauce

1 large yellow onion

2 carrots, peeled

1/2 head cauliflower, cleaned

4 tablespoons vegetable oil

2 cloves garlic, crushed

1/2 teaspoon sesame seeds

1/2 cup water

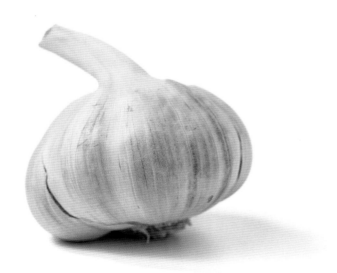

● Trim off any fat from the steak. Cut across grain into 1/8-inch strips. Put meat in a mixing bowl; add salt, 1 teaspoon of the cornstarch, and 2 teaspoons of the soy sauce. Stir to marinate meat; set aside for 30 minutes, stirring occasionally. Meanwhile, cut onion in half lengthwise; lay cut-side down and slice crosswise into 1/4-inch slices. Place onions in a separate bowl. Cut carrots in half on a long diagonal; slice on the diagonal into 1/4-inch slices. Put carrots in a separate bowl. Cut cauliflower on the diagonal into 1/4-inch slices. Add to the carrots. Heat a wok or heavy pan on high heat with 2 tablespoons of the oil. Add garlic and sesame seeds; cook 20 seconds. Add remaining oil, heat, add meat, and stir-fry quickly until brown. Remove meat from wok; keep warm. Add 1/4 cup of the water to the wok. Add onions; cook and stir 2 minutes. Add carrots and cauliflower. Stir to mix. Cover and cook just until cauliflower is crisp-tender, stirring occasionally. Combine remaining cornstarch, soy sauce, and water in a bowl or jar. Shake or stir to completely blend. Add meat to wok; stir to mix. Push meat and vegetables up side of wok. Add cornstarch mixture; cook and stir until thickened. Mix with the meat and vegetables. Pour onto hot serving platter.

EACH SERVING: ABOUT 311 CALORIES, 17 G PROTEIN, 9 G CARBOHYDRATE, 23 G TOTAL FAT (6 G SATURATED), 41 MG CHOLESTEROL, 1,405 MG SODIUM. EXCHANGE, 1 SERVING: 2/3 BREAD, 1 VEGETABLE, 3 MEDIUM-FAT MEAT

PREP TIME: 25 MINUTES COOK TIME: 20 MINUTES

Hot Spanish-Style Chorizo

MAKES 8 SERVINGS

$1/2$ cup red wine, chilled

1 tablespoon cider vinegar

1 teaspoon dark corn syrup

$1/2$ teaspoon fennel seed

1 teaspoon chili powder

$1/2$ teaspoon ground cumin

2 cloves garlic, minced

1 tablespoon onion powder

1 teaspoon ground oregano

2 teaspoons ground paprika

1 teaspoon cayenne pepper

1 teaspoon cayenne pepper flakes

$3/4$ teaspoon salt

1 pound freshly ground pork

1 cup wheat germ

• Mix wine, vinegar, and corn syrup in a large mixing bowl. Crush fennel seed in mortar with pestle. Blend seasonings into the liquid. Add pork and wheat germ. Mix sausage with clean hands until thoroughly blended. Makes 8 patties or links per recipe. Cook sausage as desired.

EACH SERVING: ABOUT 226 CALORIES, 14 G PROTEIN, 10 G CARBOHYDRATE, 14 G TOTAL FAT (5 G SATURATED), 41 MG CHOLESTEROL, 255 MG SODIUM. EXCHANGE, 1 SERVING: 2 HIGH-FAT MEAT

PREP TIME: 5 MINUTES COOK TIME: 55 MINUTES

German Goulash

MAKES 1 SERVING

3 ounces lean ground beef

1 teaspoon onion, chopped

1 tablespoon green pepper, chopped

1 tablespoon celery, chopped

$1/4$ bay leaf

$1/2$ cup kidney beans, cooked

$1/2$ cup cooked elbow macaroni

$1/4$ cup carrots, sliced

salt and pepper to taste

• Brown ground beef, onion, green pepper, and celery over low heat; drain. Add bay leaf, kidney beans, macaroni, and carrots; mix gently. Add salt and pepper. Pour into casserole dish; cover. Bake at 350°F for 40 minutes.

• Microwave: Cook on Medium for 7 minutes.

ABOUT 455 CALORIES, 27 G PROTEIN, 45 G CARBOHYDRATE, 19 G TOTAL FAT (7 G SATURATED), 64 MG CHOLESTEROL, 288 MG SODIUM. EXCHANGE: 3 MEDIUM-FAT MEAT, 2$1/2$ BREAD

Beef and Vegetable Stir-Fry

MAKES 4 SERVINGS

Feel free to pick and choose your favorite vegetables to use in this stir-fry.

$1/2$ *pound round steak, $1/2$-inch thick*

2 yellow onions

4 tomatoes

1 green pepper

$1/4$ *cup water*

1 tablespoon soy sauce

2 teaspoons cornstarch

$1/2$ *teaspoon salt*

3 tablespoons vegetable oil

1 slice gingerroot

● Cut steak across the grain into $1/8$-inch-thick and 2-inch-long strips. Slice onions, tomatoes, and green pepper into $1/2$-inch wedges. Combine water, soy sauce, cornstarch, salt, and 1 teaspoon of the oil. Stir to blend and set aside. Heat remaining oil in wok or skillet; add beef strips and the gingerroot. Stir and cook until well-browned. Add onions and stir-fry 1 minute. Add pepper and stir-fry 1 minute longer. Stir in cornstarch mixture and cook until sauce is clear. Add tomatoes and heat slightly.

EACH SERVING: ABOUT 265 CALORIES, 14 G PROTEIN, 14 G CARBOHYDRATE, 18 G TOTAL FAT (4 G SATURATED), 36 MG CHOLESTEROL, 592 MG SODIUM. EXCHANGE, 1 SERVING: 1 VEGETABLE, 2 MEDIUM-FAT MEAT, $1/2$ FAT

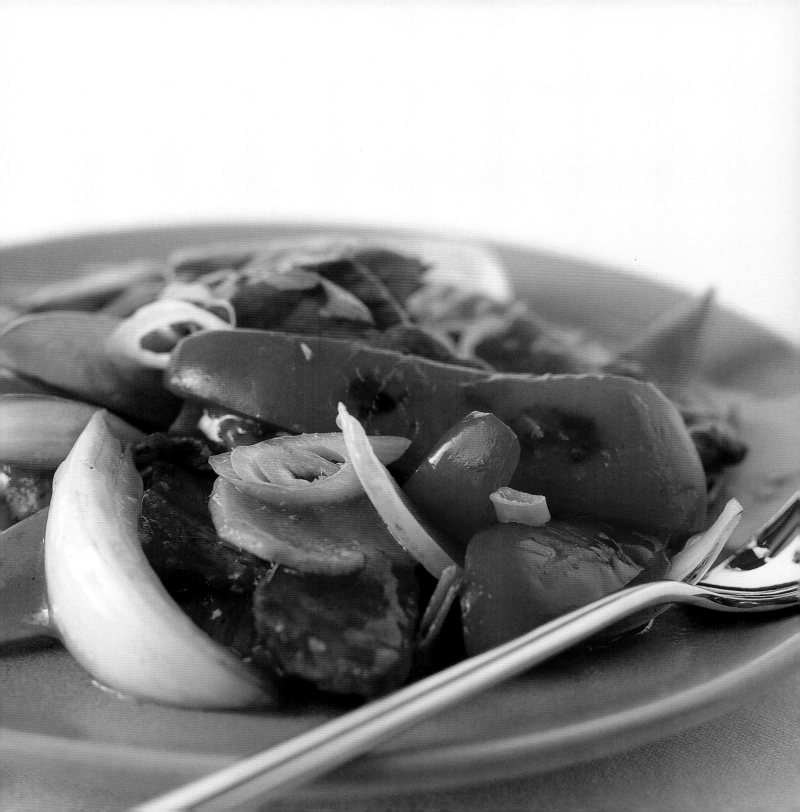

Beef and Rice Casserole

MAKES 1 SERVING

3 ounces ground beef

1 tablespoon onion, chopped

1 tablespoon celery, chopped

3/4 cups condensed chicken gumbo soup

1/4 cup water

1/2 cup uncooked rice

1/4 cup condensed cream of mushroom soup

salt and pepper to taste

● Combine ground beef, onion, and celery with a small amount of water in a saucepan. Boil until onion is tender; drain and set aside. Combine condensed chicken gumbo soup, water, and rice. Simmer until all moisture is absorbed by the rice. Mix beef mixture, rice mixture, and mushroom soup; pour into a small greased casserole dish. Add salt and pepper. Bake at 350°F for 25 minutes.

● Microwave: Cook on Medium for 8 to 10 minutes

ABOUT 722 CALORIES, 27 G PROTEIN, 94 G CARBOHYDRATE, 25 G TOTAL FAT (9 G SATURATED), 70 MG CHOLESTEROL, 1,939 MG SODIUM. EXCHANGE: 3 HIGH-FAT MEAT, 2 BREAD

Quick Kabobs

MAKES 1 SERVING

2 ounces cooked roast beef, cut in 1-inch cubes

6 1-inch-square pieces green pepper

6 cherry tomatoes

6 1-inch cubes zucchini

6 unsweetened pineapple chunks

2 tablespoons low-calorie French dressing

● Alternate beef, vegetables, and fruit on 2 skewers. Brush with 1 tablespoon of the French dressing. Broil 5 to 6 inches from heat for 8 minutes. Brush with remaining French dressing. Broil 4 minutes longer.

ABOUT 544 CALORIES, 34 G PROTEIN, 90 G CARBOHYDRATE, 12 G TOTAL FAT (4 G SATURATED), 60 MG CHOLESTEROL, 344 MG SODIUM. EXCHANGE: 2 MEDIUM-FAT MEAT, 1 VEGETABLE, 1 FRUIT

PREP TIME: 10 MINUTES   COOK TIME: 30 MINUTES

Beef Stroganoff

MAKES 1 SERVING

3 ounces lean beef, cubed

1 teaspoon margarine

1/2 onion, cut into large pieces

1/4 teaspoon garlic, minced

2 tablespoons mushroom pieces

1/2 cup condensed cream of mushroom soup

1 tablespoon low-calorie sour cream

1 teaspoon ketchup

dash Worcestershire sauce

dash salt

dash pepper

1 cup cooked noodles

• Brown beef cubes in margarine. Add onion, garlic, and mushrooms. Cook over low heat until onion is partially cooked; remove from heat. Combine condensed soup, sour cream, ketchup, Worcestershire sauce, and seasonings; blend well. Pour over beef mixture; heat thoroughly. (Do not boil.) Serve over noodles.

ABOUT 659 CALORIES, 27 G PROTEIN, 57 G CARBOHYDRATE, 36 G TOTAL FAT (12 G SATURATED), 116 MG CHOLESTEROL, 1,191 MG SODIUM. EXCHANGE: 3 HIGH-FAT MEAT, 2¹/2 BREAD

PREP TIME: 15 MINUTES   COOK TIME: 1 HOUR

Ham and Scalloped Potatoes

MAKES 1 SERVING

2 ounces lean ham, diced

1 medium potato, peeled and sliced

2 tablespoons onion

2 teaspoons parsley

1/4 cup condensed cream of celery soup

1/4 cup milk

salt and pepper to taste

• Combine ham, potato, onion, and parsley in baking dish coated with vegetable cooking spray. Blend condensed soup and milk; pour over potato mixture; cover. Bake at 350°F for 1 hour, or until potatoes are tender. Add salt and pepper.

• Microwave: Cook on high for 10 minutes, or until potatoes are tender. Add salt and pepper.

ABOUT 222 CALORIES, 16 G PROTEIN, 26 G CARBOHYDRATE, 6 G TOTAL FAT (2 G SATURATED), 35 MG CHOLESTEROL, 1,325 MG SODIUM. EXCHANGE: 2 HIGH-FAT MEAT, 1¹/2 BREAD, 1/2 MILK

Beef Becquee

MAKES 2 SERVINGS

1 cup cooked beef with fat removed

1/2 cup celery, chopped

1 small onion, chopped

1/4 cup ketchup

2 tablespoons prepared mustard

2 tablespoons water

1 tablespoon Worcestershire sauce

4 starch/bread exchanges

• Combine beef, celery, and onion in a food processor. With the steel blade, process until beef is shredded. Turn into a saucepan. Add ketchup, mustard, water, and Worcestershire sauce. Heat thoroughly. Pile on starch/bread exchanges. This is great on a hamburger bun.

EACH SERVING: ABOUT 397 CALORIES, 34 G PROTEIN, 42 G CARBOHYDRATE, 11 G TOTAL FAT (3 G SATURATED), 81 MG CHOLESTEROL, 1,422 MG SODIUM. EXCHANGE, EACH SERVING: 2 STARCH/BREAD, 3 MEDIUM-FAT MEAT

Dilly Beef

MAKES 2 SERVINGS

The dill weed in the beef adds a new taste to an old favorite.

1/4 pound ground beef

1 teaspoon dill weed

1 teaspoon ketchup

1/2 teaspoon prepared mustard

salt and pepper to taste

• Combine beef, dill weed, ketchup, mustard, salt, and pepper in a bowl. With your hands or a spoon, thoroughly blend. Form meat into two patties. Then fry in a skillet or on a grill over hot coals to desired doneness.

EACH SERVING: ABOUT 154 CALORIES, 10 G PROTEIN, 1 G CARBOHYDRATE, 12 G TOTAL FAT (5 G SATURATED), 43 MG CHOLESTEROL, 84 MG SODIUM. EXCHANGE, EACH SERVING: 1 3/4 MEDIUM-FAT MEAT

Parmigiana Ham

MAKES 1 SERVING

2 ounces ham, sliced
1 tablespoon skim milk
1 tablespoon dry bread crumbs
1 tablespoon sunflower oil
1 1/2-ounce slice of low-fat mozzarella cheese
2 tablespoons canned pizza sauce

• Dip ham slice in skim milk. Pat dry bread crumbs on both sides of the ham slice. Heat oil in skillet; then add ham slice. Brown on both sides. Top the ham slice with mozzarella cheese slice and pizza sauce. Cover and heat until cheese is melted.

ABOUT 303 CALORIES, 15 G PROTEIN, 10 G CARBOHYDRATE, 23 G TOTAL FAT (5 G SATURATED), 42 MG CHOLESTEROL, 1,064 MG SODIUM. EXCHANGE: 2 HIGH-FAT MEAT, 2 FAT, 1/3 STARCH/BREAD

Sweet and Sour Pork

MAKES 4 SERVINGS

I use an Iowa chop (a double-thick chop) for my pork cubes.

4 ounces pork cubes with fat removed
1 teaspoon soy sauce
1 tablespoon and 1 teaspoon cornstarch
2 tablespoons olive oil
1/2 onion, cut in pieces
dash ground ginger
1/4 cup pineapple chunks, in their own juice
1 tablespoon cold water
2 teaspoons white vinegar
2 teaspoons granulated sugar replacement

• Combine pork cubes and soy sauce in a bowl. Stir or toss to coat pork cubes with the soy sauce. Dredge the pork cubes in the 1 tablespoon of cornstarch, shaking off any excess. Heat the olive oil in a skillet or wok. Brown the pork cubes. Add the onion and ground ginger. Stir-fry until onions are soft. Add pineapple chunks and juice. While stirring, cook for 1 minute. Combine water, vinegar, sugar replacement, and the 1 teaspoon of cornstarch in shaker bottle; then shake to mix. Pour over pork cubes. While stirring, cook until mixture becomes clear and thickens.

EACH SERVING: ABOUT 145 CALORIES, 9 G PROTEIN, 6 G CARBOHYDRATE, 10 G TOTAL FAT (2 G SATURATED), 24 MG CHOLESTEROL, 103 MG SODIUM. EXCHANGE, EACH SERVING: 1 LEAN MEAT, 1 FAT, 1/4 STARCH/BREAD

PREP TIME: 20 MINUTES   COOK TIME: 30 MINUTES

Curried Meatballs

MAKES 4 SERVINGS

MEATBALLS:

1/2 pound lean ground beef

2 tablespoons chopped onion

1 small clove garlic, minced

2 teaspoons all-purpose flour

dash each allspice, salt, and pepper

2 tablespoons vegetable oil

CURRY SAUCE:

1 tablespoon low-calorie margarine

1/2 cup finely chopped onion

1/2 teaspoon garlic powder

2 teaspoons curry powder

1/2 cup water

1 cube chicken bouillon

2 teaspoons tomato paste

To make meatballs:

● Combine beef, onion, garlic, flour, and seasonings in a bowl. With your hands or a spoon, mix to blend thoroughly. Form into small walnut-size balls. Heat oil in a skillet. Brown meatballs on all sides. Remove meatballs from skillet.

To make curry sauce:

● Melt margarine in skillet. Add onion and garlic powder. While stirring, cook over low heat until onions are soft. Stir in curry powder. Add remaining ingredients. Stir to dissolve bouillon cube and blend mixture. Add meatballs. Cover and simmer for 10 minutes.

EACH SERVING: ABOUT 249 CALORIES, 11 G PROTEIN, 5 G CARBOHYDRATE, 21 G TOTAL FAT (6 G SATURATED), 43 MG CHOLESTEROL, 283 MG SODIUM. EXCHANGE, EACH SERVING: 13/4 HIGH-FAT MEAT

Beef Beauties

MAKES 4 SERVINGS

1 cup cooked beef with fat removed
1/2 cup sliced celery
1/4 onion
1 teaspoon Dijon mustard
4 starch/bread exchanges
pimiento, if desired

● Combine beef, celery, onion, and mustard in food processor. With its steel blade, process the mixture until the meat is finely shredded. (If you don't have a food processor, finely chop the ingredients.) Pile beef mixture on two starch/bread exchanges. Top each sandwich with another starch/bread exchange. Cut in half. For appetizers, cut four starch/bread exchanges into four squares; then divide beef mixture evenly among the 16 squares. If desired, top each appetizer with a slice of pimiento.

EACH SERVING: ABOUT 230 CALORIES, 14 G PROTEIN, 14 G CARBOHYDRATE, 13 G TOTAL FAT (5 G SATURATED), 40 MG CHOLESTEROL, 199 MG SODIUM. EXCHANGE, EACH SERVING: 1 STARCH/BREAD, 1¹/2 MEDIUM-FAT MEAT

Pile-High Porkies

MAKES 2 SERVINGS

1 cup cooked pork with fat removed
1/3 cup green onion, chopped
1/4 cup carrot, chopped
2 tablespoons Dijon mustard
2 hamburger rolls, split
1/4 cup Cheddar cheese, shredded

● Combine pork, green onion, carrot, and mustard in a food processor. With the steel blade, process until meat is shredded. Under the broiler, toast the bottom half of each roll. Divide pork mixture evenly between the two toasted bottom halves. Sprinkle Cheddar cheese on top of pork mixture. Place sandwich on broiler pan. Place top halves of rolls on broiler pan, with top sides down. Then place under broiler until cheese is melted and insides of top halves of rolls are golden brown.

EACH SERVING: ABOUT 368 CALORIES, 34 G PROTEIN, 25 G CARBOHYDRATE, 14 G TOTAL FAT (6 G SATURATED), 96 MG CHOLESTEROL, 420 MG SODIUM. EXCHANGE, EACH SERVING: 3¹/2 HIGH-FAT MEAT, 2 STARCH/BREAD

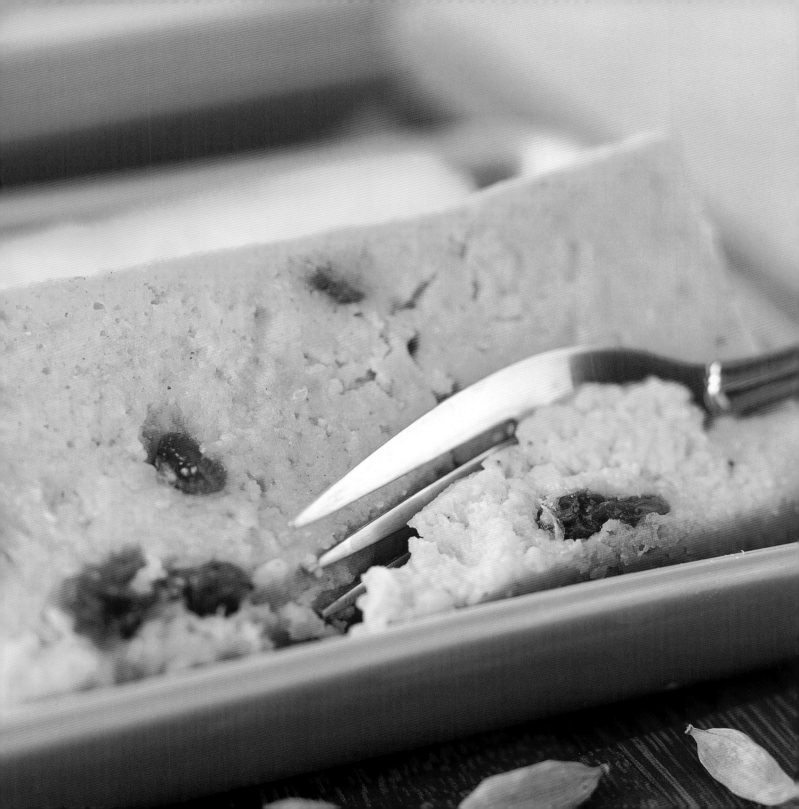

Breads & Baked Goods

Bran Bread •

Jewish Braid Bread (Challah) •

Quick Onion Bread •

Apricot Bread •

Strawberry Banana Muffins •

French Toast Torrijas •

Raisin Bread •

Pita Bread •

Pioneer Cornbread •

Baking Powder Biscuits •

Orange Muffins •

Fresh Apple Muffins •

Sunday Morning Scones •

• Rosemary Raisin Buns

• Haitian Sweet Potato Bread

• Vilpuri Twist

• Irish Soda Bread

• Tea Scones

• Popovers

• Lemon Buns

• Blue-Cheese Bread

• Orange Bread

• Graham Bread

• Chocolate Bread

• Amaretto Tea Bread

• Quick French Bread

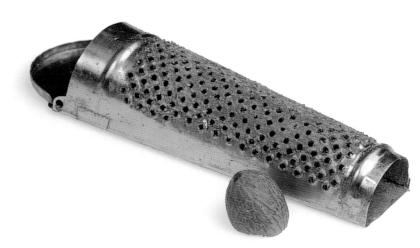

PREP TIME: 40 MINUTES COOK TIME: 50 TO 55 MINUTES
(LET RISE 3 HOURS)

Bran Bread

MAKES 1 LOAF (14 SLICES)

3 tablespoons shortening

3 tablespoons brown sugar replacement

3 tablespoons molasses

1 teaspoon salt

1/2 cup bran

3/4 cup boiling water

1 package dry yeast

1/4 cup warm water

2 1/2 cups flour

margarine, melted

● Place shortening, brown sugar replacement, molasses, salt, and bran in large mixing bowl. Add boiling water. Stir to blend. Dissolve dry yeast in warm water. Allow to rest for 5 minutes. Add yeast to bran mixture. Add flour, 1 cup at a time, stirring well between additions, until a soft dough is formed. Knead gently for 10 minutes. Shape into loaf. Place in greased 13" x 9" x 2" loaf pan. Cover; allow to rise for 2 hours. Punch down; allow to rise for 1 hour. Bake at 325°F for 50 to 55 minutes. Remove to rack and brush lightly with melted margarine.

EACH SLICE: ABOUT 123 CALORIES, 3 G PROTEIN, 22 G CARBOHYDRATE,
3 G TOTAL FAT (1 G SATURATED), 0 MG CHOLESTEROL, 167 MG SODIUM.
EXCHANGE, 1 SLICE: 1 BREAD

PREP TIME: 40 MINUTES COOK TIME: 1 HOUR
(LET RISE 3 HOURS)

Jewish Braid Bread (Challah)

MAKES 1 LOAF (18 SLICES)

1 package dry yeast

3/4 cup warm water

1 teaspoon salt

1/4 cup sugar replacement

2 tablespoons margarine, melted

2 eggs, well beaten

3 cups flour

1 teaspoon skim milk

poppy seeds

● Soften yeast in warm water; allow to rest for 5 minutes. Add salt, sugar replacement, and margarine. Measure 1 tablespoon of the beaten eggs. Place in cup and reserve. Add remaining eggs and 1 cup of the flour to yeast mixture; beat vigorously. Add remaining flour. Turn onto floured board and knead until smooth and elastic. Place in lightly greased bowl; cover. Allow to rise until double in size, about 1 1/2 hours. Punch down; divide into thirds. Roll into three 18-inch strips, with the heel of the hand. Braid the three strips loosely, tucking under ends. Blend reserved beaten egg with 1 teaspoon skim milk; carefully brush over braid. Sprinkle with poppy seeds; cover. Allow to rise until double in size, about 1 1/2 hours. Bake at 350°F for 1 hour, or until done.

EACH SLICE: ABOUT 97 CALORIES, 3 G PROTEIN, 16 G CARBOHYDRATE,
2 G TOTAL FAT (TRACE SATURATED), 24 MG CHOLESTEROL, 153 MG SODIUM.
EXCHANGE, 1 SLICE: 1 BREAD

Quick Onion Bread

MAKES 1 LOAF (14 SLICES)

1 loaf frozen bread dough

1 package onion soup mix

● Allow bread to thaw as directed on package. Roll dough out on unfloured board. Sprinkle half of soup mix over surface. Roll up jelly-roll style. Knead to work mix into dough; repeat with remaining soup mix. Form into loaf. Place in greased 9" x 5" loaf pan; cover. Allow to rise about 2 hours. Bake at 350°F for 30 to 40 minutes, or until done.

EACH SLICE: ABOUT 129 CALORIES, 4 G PROTEIN, 24 G CARBOHYDRATE, 3 G FAT (TRACE SATURATED), 0 MG CHOLESTEROL, 205 MG SODIUM. EXCHANGE, 1 SLICE: 1 BREAD

Apricot Bread

MAKES 1 LOAF (14 SLICES)

8 dried apricot halves

1/3 cup shortening

1/4 cup brown sugar replacement, packed

2 eggs, beaten

1 cup skim milk

1/2 teaspoon salt

1 1/2 teaspoons baking powder

1/4 teaspoon cinnamon

dash nutmeg dash

3/4 cup flour

● Soak apricots in warm water for 2 hours. Cook over medium heat for 10 minutes; drain, and chop finely. Cream shortening and brown sugar replacement. Add eggs and skim milk; beat thoroughly. Add salt, baking powder, cinnamon, and nutmeg. Stir in apricots and flour to make a thick cake batter. Pour into greased 9" x 5" loaf pan. Bake at 350°F for 1 1/2 hours, or until toothpick comes out clean.

EACH SLICE: ABOUT 88 CALORIES, 2 G PROTEIN, 8 G CARBOHYDRATE, 5 G FAT (1 G SATURATED), 31 MG CHOLESTEROL, 211 MG SODIUM. EXCHANGE, 1 SLICE: 1 BREAD, 1 FAT

Strawberry Banana Muffins

MAKES 12 MUFFINS

2 cups biscuit mix

1/4 cup granulated sugar replacement

3/4 cup skim milk

2 tablespoons margarine, melted

12 medium fresh strawberries

2 small bananas

● Combine biscuit mix, sugar replacement, milk, and margarine in a medium mixing bowl. Stir to mix. (Batter will be lumpy.) Cut strawberries and bananas into small cube-like pieces. Stir into batter. Line 12 large muffin cups with paper liners. Divide batter evenly among the muffin cups. Bake at 400°F for 20 to 25 minutes or until toothpick inserted in muffin comes out clean.

EACH MUFFIN: ABOUT 112 CALORIES, 2 G PROTEIN, 15 G CARBOHYDRATE, 5 G TOTAL FAT (1 G SATURATED), 3 MG CHOLESTEROL, 172 MG SODIUM. EXCHANGE, 1 SERVING: 1¹/3 BREAD

French Toast Torrijas

MAKES 8 SERVINGS

French toast is a favorite Spanish dessert.

1 cup lowfat 1% milk

1/2 teaspoon cinnamon

8 slices white bread

2 large eggs or equivalent egg substitute,
   lightly beaten

dollop fruit jam

● Mix together milk and cinnamon in a shallow bowl. Briefly soak each slice of bread in the cinnamon milk, then dip in the beaten egg or egg substitute. Fry until brown in a hot griddle or frying pan sprayed with nonstick cooking spray. Serve immediately with jam.

EACH SERVING: ABOUT 106 CALORIES, 5 G PROTEIN, 16 G CARBOHYDRATE, 3 G FAT (1 G SATURATED), 55 MG CHOLESTEROL, 167 MG SODIUM. EXCHANGE, 1 SERVING: 1 STARCH

French Toast Torrijas

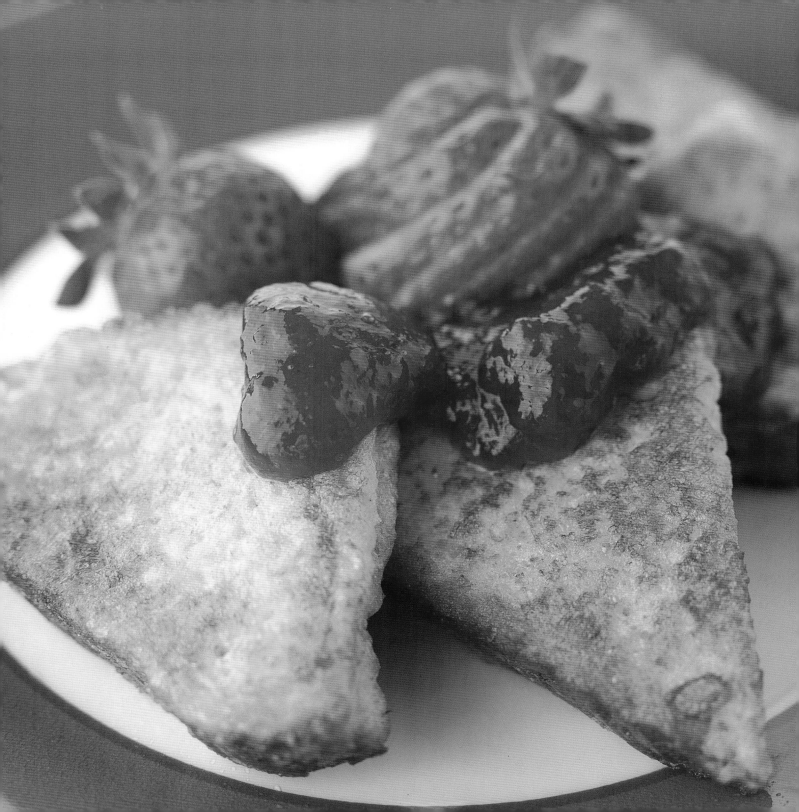

Raisin Bread

MAKES 1 LOAF (14 SLICES)

1 package dry yeast

¹/4 cup warm water

³/4 cups milk, scalded and cooled

2 tablespoons sugar replacement

1 teaspoon salt

1 egg

2 tablespoons margarine, softened

3³/4 cups flour

1 cup raisins

● Dissolve yeast in warm water; allow to rest for 5 minutes. Combine milk, sugar replacement, salt, egg, and margarine; mix thoroughly. Stir in yeast mixture. Add 1 cup of the flour. Beat until smooth. Mix in raisins. Blend in remaining flour. Knead for 5 minutes. Cover; allow to rise for 2 hours. Punch down; form into loaf. Place in greased 9" x 5" loaf pan; cover. Allow to rise for 1 hour. Bake at 400°F for 30 minutes, or until loaf sounds hollow and is golden brown. Remove to rack.

**EACH SLICE: ABOUT 181 CALORIES, 5 G PROTEIN, 35 G CARBOHYDRATE,
3 G FAT (1 G SATURATED), 16 MG CHOLESTEROL, 200 MG SODIUM.
EXCHANGE, 1 SLICE: 1 BREAD**

Pita Bread

MAKES 15 PITA BREADS

1 package dry yeast

¹/2 teaspoon sugar replacement

1 teaspoon salt

1 tablespoon liquid shortening

1¹/2 cups warm water

4 cups flour

● Dissolve yeast, sugar replacement, salt, and liquid shortening in warm water. Add 3 cups of the flour; stir to mix well. (Dough should be fairly stiff; if not, add more flour.) Turn out onto floured surface; knead in remaining flour. (Dough will be very stiff.) Form into 15¹/2-inch tube. Cut into 15 slices. Pat to make circles about 6 inches in diameter. Lay on lightly greased baking pans; cover. Allow to rise until almost doubled, about 1¹/2 to 2 hours. Bake at 475°F for 10 to 12 minutes, or until lightly golden brown, puffed, and hollow. These freeze well.

**EACH PITA BREAD: ABOUT 132 CALORIES, 4 G PROTEIN, 26 G CARBOHYDRATE,
1 G TOTAL FAT (TRACE SATURATED), 0 MG CHOLESTEROL, 155 MG SODIUM.
EXCHANGE, 1 PITA: 1¹/2 BREAD, ¹/2 FAT**

Pioneer Cornbread

MAKES 9 SQUARES

1 egg

1 cup skim milk

2 tablespoons low-calorie maple syrup

2 tablespoons margarine, melted

²/3 cups cornmeal

³/4 cup flour

1 tablespoon baking powder

1 teaspoon salt

● Beat egg until light and lemon colored. Add skim milk, maple syrup, and margarine. Combine cornmeal, flour, baking powder, and salt in large bowl. Stir to blend. Gradually add flour mixture to liquid. Pour into greased 8-inch square pan. Bake at 425°F for 20 to 25 minutes.

● Microwave: Bake on Low for 10 minutes. Increase heat to High for 5 minutes, or until toothpick comes out clean.

EACH SQUARE: ABOUT 123 CALORIES, 4 G PROTEIN, 18 G CARBOHYDRATE, 4 G TOTAL FAT (1 G SATURATED), 25 MG CHOLESTEROL, 442 MG SODIUM. EXCHANGE, 1 SQUARE: 1¹/2 BREAD

Baking Powder Biscuits

MAKES 10 BISCUITS

1 cup flour

1 teaspoon baking powder

¹/4 teaspoon yeast

¹/4 teaspoon salt

1 tablespoon liquid shortening

6 tablespoons milk

● Combine all ingredients; mix just until blended. Turn out on floured board. Roll out to a ¹/2-inch thickness. Cut into circles with floured 2-inch cutter. Place on baking sheet coated with vegetable cooking spray; cover. Allow to rest for 10 minutes. Bake at 450°F for 12 to 15 minutes, or until lightly browned.

EACH BISCUIT: ABOUT 62 CALORIES, 2 G PROTEIN, 10 G CARBOHYDRATE, 2 G TOTAL FAT (TRACE SATURATED), 0 MG CHOLESTEROL, 112 MG SODIUM. EXCHANGE, 1 BISCUIT: 1 BREAD, ¹/2 FAT

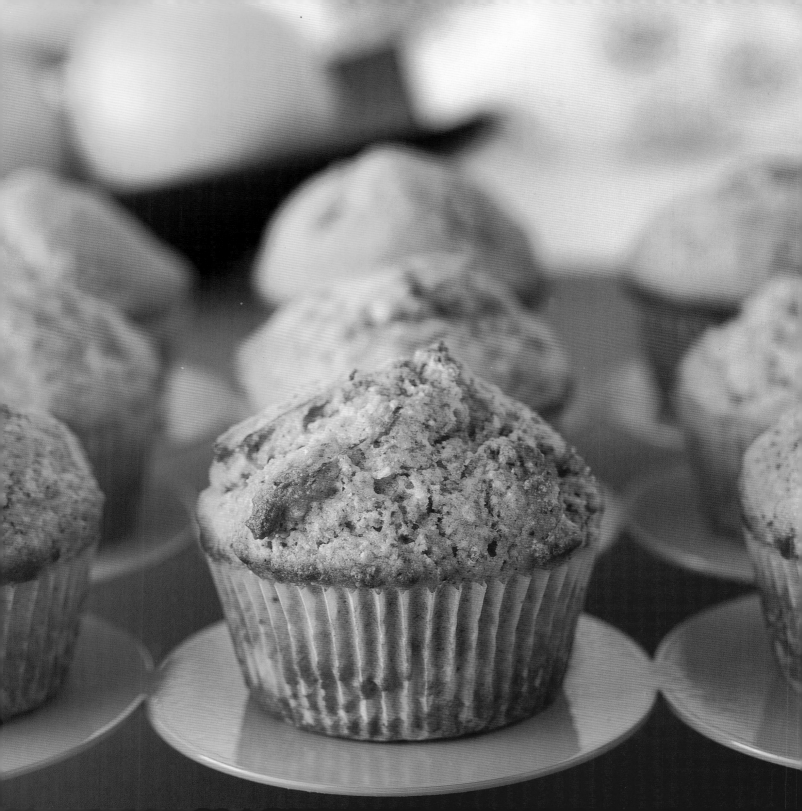

PREP TIME: 20 MINUTES   COOK TIME: 20 TO 25 MINUTES
(LET REST 1 HOUR)

Orange Muffins

MAKES 24 MUFFINS

1 cup orange juice

1 tablespoon orange peel, grated

1/2 cup raisins, soaked

1/3 cup sugar replacement

1 tablespoon margarine

1 egg

1/4 teaspoon salt

1 teaspoon baking soda

1 teaspoon baking powder

1/2 teaspoon vanilla extract

2 cups flour

● Combine orange juice, orange peel, and raisins. Allow to rest for 1 hour. Cream together the sugar replacement, margarine, and egg. Add salt, baking soda, baking powder, and vanilla extract. Stir in orange juice mixture. Stir in the flour to make a thick cake batter. Spoon into greased muffin tins, filling no more than two-thirds full. Bake at 350°F for 20 to 25 minutes, or until done.

● Microwave: Spoon into 6-ounce custard cups, filling no more than two-thirds full. Cook on Low for 7 to 8 minutes. Increase heat to High for 2 minutes, or until done.

EACH MUFFIN: ABOUT 59 CALORIES, 2 G PROTEIN, 12 G CARBOHYDRATE, 1 G TOTAL FAT (TRACE SATURATED), 9 MG CHOLESTEROL, 107 MG SODIUM. EXCHANGE, 1 MUFFIN: 1 BREAD

Orange Muffins

PREP TIME: 20 MINUTES   COOK TIME: 25 MINUTES

Fresh Apple Muffins

MAKES 12 MUFFINS

2 tablespoons soft margarine

2 tablespoons sugar replacement

1 egg, beaten

1 1/4 cups flour

1/4 teaspoon salt

2 teaspoons baking powder

6 tablespoons skim milk

1 small apple, peeled and chopped

● Cream margarine and sugar replacement; add egg. Stir in remaining ingredients. Spoon into greased muffin tins, filling no more than two-thirds full. Bake at 400°F for 25 minutes, or until done.

EACH MUFFIN: ABOUT 81 CALORIES, 2G PROTEIN, 12 G CARBOHYDRATE, 3 G TOTAL FAT (1 G SATURATED), 18 MG CHOLESTEROL, 212 MG SODIUM. EXCHANGE, 1 MUFFIN: 1 BREAD

PREP TIME: 30 MINUTES   COOK TIME: 10 MINUTES

Sunday Morning Scones

MAKES 12 SCONES

Our friends Bobby and Annette Donovan love these scones better than any others. They stopped by one Sunday morning and were fans of these after just one bite.

2 cups all-purpose flour

1 tablespoon active baker's yeast

1/2 teaspoon salt

1 tablespoon sugar

4 tablespoons butter

3 medium eggs or equivalent egg substitute

1/3 cup and 1 tablespoon lowfat 1% milk

● Combine the first four ingredients in a mixing bowl and mix well. Cut in the butter, using two knives or a pastry blender. Make a well in this mixture. Beat together the two eggs and 1/3 cup milk and add to the flour mixture. Mix lightly but thoroughly. Turn the dough out onto a lightly floured surface and knead for 5 minutes. Roll into a 9-inch circle approximately 3/4-inch thick. Cut into 12 pie-shaped wedges. Place the wedges onto a greased baking sheet. Beat together the remaining egg and 1 tablespoon milk. Brush the tops of the scones with this mixture. Bake in a preheated 400°F oven for 7 to 10 minutes. Split scones. Serve with jam or jelly made without sugar, if desired.

EACH SCONE: ABOUT 139 CALORIES, 4 G PROTEIN, 18 G CARBOHYDRATE, 5 G TOTAL FAT (3 G SATURATED), 64 MG CHOLESTEROL, 156 MG SODIUM. EXCHANGE, EACH SCONE: 1 STARCH, 1 FAT

PREP TIME: 40 MINUTES   COOK TIME: 15 TO 20 MINUTES
(LET RISE 2 HOURS)

Rosemary Raisin Buns

MAKES 16 BUNS

Most big supermarkets have fresh rosemary in the produce section. When you have fresh rosemary, make these buns. They are well worth the effort.

4 heaping cups raisins
2¹/2 cups warm water
2 packets active dry yeast
2 tablespoons sugar
4 tablespoons olive oil
1 teaspoon salt
3³/4 cups flour
2 teaspoons fresh rosemary sprigs, chopped

• Put the raisins in a small bowl and pour the warm water over them. Stir to combine and set aside for 20 minutes. Drain the raisins, saving 1¹/4 cup of the raisin water to be used now, and save the rest of the raisin water to use later as a glaze. In a small saucepan, warm the 1¹/4 cups of raisin water in a small saucepan to about 105°F to 115°F. Combine this heated water with the yeast in a large mixing bowl. Set aside for 10 minutes. The yeast should bubble and become creamy. Stir in the sugar and 2 tablespoons of olive oil. Stir in the salt. Add the flour gradually, mixing until the dough is no longer sticky. Turn onto a lightly floured work surface and knead until smooth and elastic.

• Place the dough in an oiled bowl, cover with a tea towel or plastic wrap, and set to rise in a warm, draft-free place for an hour or until doubled in size.

• Put the remaining 2 tablespoons of olive oil in a small frying pan and sauté the rosemary leaves and the drained raisins. Stir constantly. Cool. The raisins will be plump.

• Punch down the dough and turn onto a lightly floured work surface. Shape the dough into a large rectangle. Sprinkle the rosemary mixture over the dough and roll up, jelly-roll style. Cover with a tea towel or plastic wrap for 10 minutes.

• Shape the dough into 16 balls. Place the balls on lightly oiled cookie sheets. Cover with the towel and let rise for a second time for about an hour.

• With a fork, prick a cross on the top of each bun. Reshape the buns into balls with your fingers, if needed. Brush on a glaze of reserved raisin water. Cover with a towel again while the oven preheats to 400°F. Bake for 15 to 20 minutes. Buns will be golden. Remove to racks to cool.

EACH BUN: ABOUT 168 CALORIES, 4 G PROTEIN, 30 G CARBOHYDRATE, 4 G TOTAL FAT (1 G SATURATED), 0 MG CHOLESTEROL, 147 MG SODIUM. EXCHANGE, EACH BUN: 1 STARCH, 1 FRUIT

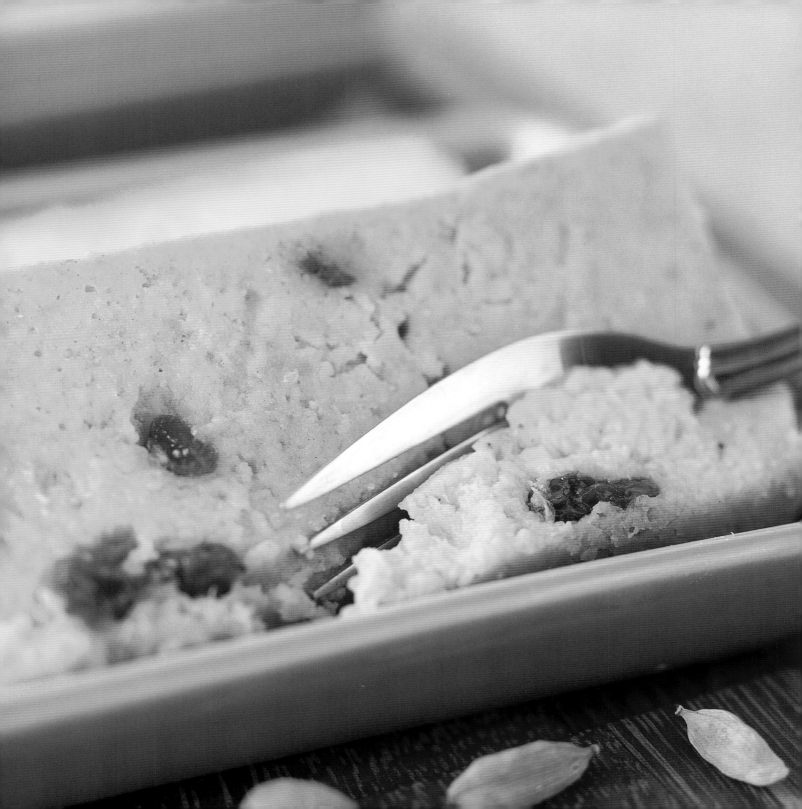

PREP TIME: 30 MINUTES   COOK TIME: 1 HOUR 30 MINUTES

Haitian Sweet Potato Bread

MAKES 1 LOAF (20 SLICES)

There may be no flour, but this "bread" is moist and smooth.

2 pounds sweet potatoes, peeled and cut in quarters

1 large ripe banana, peeled and cut into 1-inch
   chunks

4 tablespoons butter

3 large eggs or equivalent egg substitute, lightly
   beaten

$1/4$ cup sugar

$1/4$ cup dark corn syrup

$1/2$ cup lowfat 1% milk

$1/2$ cup evaporated milk

$1/2$ teaspoon vanilla extract

$1/4$ teaspoon ground nutmeg

$1/4$ teaspoon ground cinnamon

$1/4$ cup seedless raisins

● Bring a pot of water to a boil and drop in the sweet potatoes. Cook briskly until soft. Drain the sweet potatoes. Purée the banana and potatoes. Transfer to a mixing bowl. Beat in the butter and eggs. Add the remaining ingredients. Pour the batter into a well-greased 9" x 5" x 3" bread pan. Bake in a preheated 350°F oven for $1^{1}/2$ hours. When done, a cake tester in the center will come out clean. The top will be golden brown. Cool for about 5 minutes. Turn out onto a wire rack to cool completely.

EACH SLICE: ABOUT 134 CALORIES, 23 G CARBOHYDRATE, 4 G TOTAL FAT
(2 G SATURATED), 40 MG CHOLESTEROL, 54 MG SODIUM.
EXCHANGE, EACH SLICE: 1 STARCH, 1 FAT

PREP TIME: 40 MINUTES   COOK TIME: 20 MINUTES
(LET RISE 1 HOUR 30 MINUTES TO 2 HOURS 15 MINUTES)

Vilpuri Twist

MAKES 3 LOAVES (60 SLICES)

Cardamom gives a traditional flavor to this coffee bread. This dough is a delight to work with.

5¹/2 cups all-purpose flour

2 packages active baker's yeast

¹/2 teaspoon ground cardamom

¹/2 teaspoon ground nutmeg

2 cups lowfat 1% milk

¹/2 cup sugar substitute

¹/4 cup butter, margarine, or fat-free replacement

1 teaspoon salt

2 large eggs, at room temperature, or egg substitute, lightly beaten

1 tablespoon water

● In a large mixing bowl combine 2¹/2 cups flour with the yeast, cardamom, and nutmeg. In a saucepan, heat together the milk, sugar substitute, butter, and salt just until warm. Add to the dry mixture. Add 1 egg. With an electric mixer, beat for a minute at a low speed, until thoroughly moistened, scraping the bowl constantly. Beat for 3 minutes at high speed. By hand, beat in enough of the remaining flour to make a stiff dough. Turn onto a floured work surface. Knead until smooth and elastic. Place in a greased bowl and turn once to grease the surface. Cover with a tea towel or plastic wrap. Let rise in a warm place until double in bulk, for 1 to 1¹/2 hours.

● Punch down. Divide into thirds and let rest for 10 minutes. On a lightly floured work surface, shape one-third of the dough into a rope at least 36 inches long. Form the dough rope into a circle with a 6-inch overlap on the two ends closest to you. Holding the ends of the dough rope toward the center of the circle, twist together twice. Press the ends together and tuck under the center of the top of the circle, forming a pretzel-shaped roll. Place on a well-greased baking sheet. Repeat with the remaining dough to make three twists. Let each rise until almost double in bulk (30 to 45 minutes). Bake twists in a preheated 375°F oven about 20 minutes. The breads will be light and will sound hollow when tapped. Beat the remaining egg with water. Brush the egg mixture on the hot breads. Makes three loaves.

EACH SLICE: ABOUT 62 CALORIES, 2 G PROTEIN, 11 G CARBOHYDRATE,
1 G TOTAL FAT (1 G SATURATED), 10 MG CHOLESTEROL, 53 MG SODIUM.
EXCHANGE, EACH SLICE: 1 STARCH

Irish Soda Bread

MAKES 20 SERVINGS

This traditional Irish quick bread is served in the late afternoon with tea. It all goes together easily, and you'll love having the smell of homemade bread baking in your home.

4 cups all-purpose flour, sifted

2 tablespoons sugar

1 teaspoon active baker's yeast

1 teaspoon salt

1 cup seedless raisins

1 cup fat-free buttermilk*

1 teaspoon butter or equivalent butter substitute,
*   softened*

*Or substitute with 1 cup lowfat milk and 1 tablespoon vinegar.

● Combine the first five ingredients in a mixing bowl and stir well. Make a well in the center. Add buttermilk. Stir until lightly but thoroughly blended. Use only enough buttermilk to make a stiff dough. Turn out onto a lightly floured work surface and knead only five times. Form into a ball and place on a lightly greased cookie sheet. Pat into an 8-inch circle, approximately 1^{1}/2-inches thick.

● With a floured knife, cut a large cross on top of the loaf. Spread the top of the loaf with butter. Bake in a preheated 375°F oven 40 to 50 minutes or until golden. Serve hot, with jam or jelly.

EACH SERVING: ABOUT 124 CALORIES, 3 G PROTEIN, 27 G CARBOHYDRATE, TRACE FAT (TRACE SATURATED), 1 MG CHOLESTEROL, 123 MG SODIUM. EXCHANGE, EACH SERVING: 1 STARCH, 1 FRUIT

PREP TIME: 35 MINUTES   COOK TIME: 15 MINUTES

Tea Scones

MAKES 8 SCONES

1 cup flour

1 teaspoon baking powder

¹/4 teaspoon salt

1 tablespoon sugar replacement

¹/4 cup cold margarine

1 egg

¹/4 cup evaporated skim milk

● Sift together flour, baking powder, salt, and sugar replacement. Cut in cold margarine as for pie crust. Beat egg and evaporated milk together thoroughly; stir into flour mixture. Knead gently on lightly floured board. Divide dough in half; roll each half into a circle. Cut circles into quarters. Place on lightly greased cookie sheet. Brush tops with milk. Bake at 450°F for 15 minutes, or until done.

EACH SCONE: ABOUT 124 CALORIES, 3 G PROTEIN, 13 G CARBOHYDRATE, 7 G TOTAL FAT (1 G SATURATED), 27 MG CHOLESTEROL, 227 MG SODIUM. EXCHANGE, 1 SCONE: 1 BREAD

PREP TIME: 20 MINUTES   COOK TIME: 50 MINUTES

Popovers

MAKES 18 POPOVERS

1 cup flour

¹/2 teaspoon salt

2 eggs

1 cup skim milk

● Sift flour and salt together; set aside. Beat eggs and skim milk; add to flour. Beat until smooth and creamy. Pour into heated greased muffin tins, filling half full or less. Bake at 375°F for 50 minutes, or until popovers are golden brown and sound hollow. Do not open oven for first 40 minutes.

EACH POPOVER: ABOUT 34 CALORIES, 1 G PROTEIN, 5 G CARBOHYDRATE, 1 G TOTAL FAT (TRACE SATURATED), 24 MG CHOLESTEROL, 71 MG SODIUM. EXCHANGE, 1 POPOVER: ¹/2 BREAD, ¹/8 MEAT

Popovers

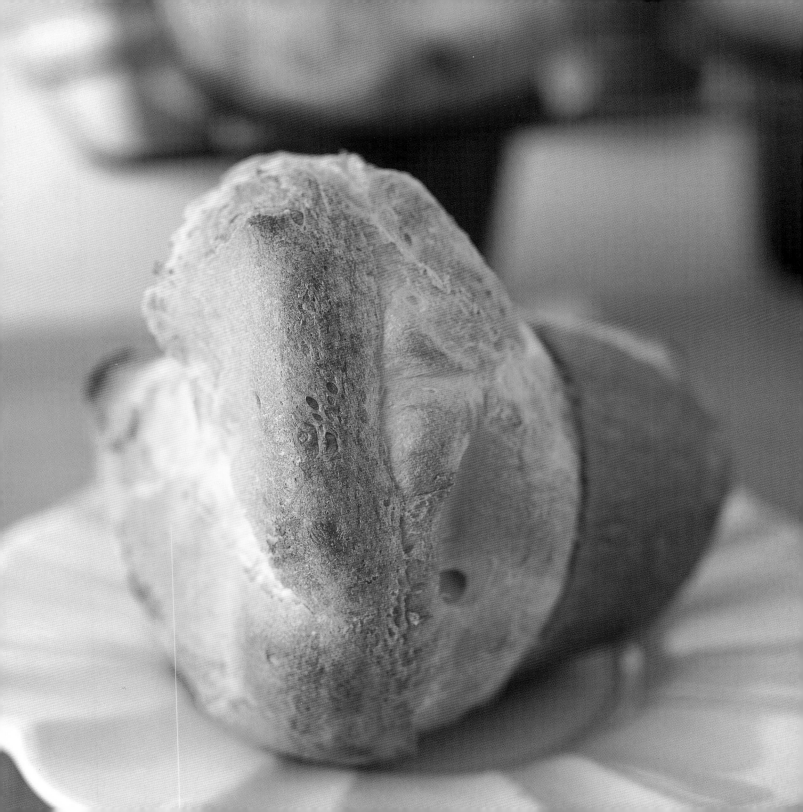

PREP TIME: 30 MINUTES   COOK TIME: 10 MINUTES
(LET RISE 2 HOURS)

Lemon Buns

MAKES 24 BUNS

These are light and flavorful: perfect with espresso or fancy coffee.

2 packets active baker's yeast

3/4 cup lowfat 1% milk

3 1/2 cups flour

1/4 cup sugar substitute

1 teaspoon salt

1/3 cup olive oil

2 large eggs or equivalent egg substitute, lightly beaten

2 teaspoons lemon peel, grated

1 teaspoon lemon extract

1 teaspoon vanilla extract

1 large egg white, beaten

● Put the yeast into a small bowl. Heat the milk in a small saucepan to 105°F to 115°F. Pour over the yeast. Stir. Let stand for 10 minutes. The yeast should bubble and become creamy. Add 1/2 cup of the flour. Stir. Cover with a tea towel or plastic wrap. Set in a warm, draft-free place for 20 minutes. The mixture should double. Place the remaining flour, sugar substitute, and salt into a large mixing bowl. Stir in the yeast mixture, olive oil, eggs, lemon peel, and extracts. Knead on a lightly floured work surface until smooth, adding more flour if needed. The dough inside will stay sticky. Place the dough in a lightly oiled bowl, cover with a tea towel or plastic wrap, and let rise for 1 to 2 hours, until doubled. Turn the dough out onto the lightly floured work surface and cut into 24 pieces. Roll each into a ball. Place them on lightly oiled cookie sheets. Cover with a tea towel or plastic wrap and let rise one hour, until doubled. Glaze each of the buns with the beaten egg white. Bake in a preheated 325°F oven for 10 minutes. The buns should be golden and not too brown on the bottom. Remove to racks to cool.

EACH BUN: ABOUT 116 CALORIES, 3 G PROTEIN, 17 G CARBOHYDRATE,
4 G TOTAL FAT (1 G SATURATED), 18 MG CHOLESTEROL, 109 MG SODIUM.
EXCHANGE, EACH BUN: 1 STARCH, 1 FAT

Blue-Cheese Bread

MAKES 2 LOAVES (24 SERVINGS)

1 envelope yeast

1 teaspoon granulated sugar

1/4 cup warm water

3/4 cup skim milk

1/4 cup blue cheese

1/4 cup finely chopped chives

1 tablespoon sunflower oil

2 1/2 cups bread flour

1/2 cup rye flour

● Sprinkle yeast and sugar over warm water in bowl. Allow to soften; then stir to dissolve. In a blender, combine milk and blue cheese. Blend on high until mixture is creamy. Pour into a large mixing bowl. Stir in yeast-sugar mixture, chives, and oil. Add half the bread flour; then beat into a batter. Continue beating, gradually adding remaining bread flour and the rye flour. Cover and allow to rise until doubled in size. Now grease two 8-inch baking pans. Divide dough in half. Form each half of the dough into the bottom of the baking pans. Cover and allow to rise until doubled in size. Bake at 400°F for 30 minutes or until done. Then immediately remove from pans and allow to cool on racks.

**EACH SERVING: ABOUT 76 CALORIES, 3 G PROTEIN, 13 G CARBOHYDRATE,
1 G FAT (TRACE SATURATED), 1 MG CHOLESTEROL, 24 MG SODIUM.
EXCHANGE, 1 SERVING: 3/4 STARCH/BREAD**

Orange Bread

MAKES 16 SERVINGS

This bread is especially good with ham.

1 cup orange juice

1 envelope dry yeast

1 tablespoon low-calorie margarine, melted

1 teaspoon honey

1 teaspoon salt

1 teaspoon grated orange rind

3 cups all-purpose flour

● Heat orange juice until lukewarm. Stir in yeast, margarine, and honey. Allow yeast to soften; then stir to dissolve completely. Add salt and orange rind. Next, add flour. Mix well. Allow to rise until doubled in size. Turn out onto lightly floured board; then knead for 10 minutes. Form into a loaf. Place in lightly oiled loaf pan. Cover and allow to rise. Bake at 375°F for 30 to 40 minutes.

**EACH SERVING: ABOUT 99 CALORIES, 3 G PROTEIN, 20 G CARBOHYDRATE,
1 G TOTAL FAT (TRACE SATURATED), 0 MG CHOLESTEROL, 154 MG SODIUM.
EXCHANGE, EACH SERVING: 1 STARCH/BREAD**

PREP TIME: 15 MINUTES   COOK TIME: 50 MINUTES
(LET RISE 2 HOURS)

Graham Bread

MAKES 2 LOAVES (30 SERVINGS)

1 envelope yeast

1/4 cup lukewarm water

2 teaspoons honey

2 cups warm water

1/4 cup granulated brown-sugar replacement

2 tablespoons vegetable oil

2 teaspoons salt

1/2 cup all-purpose flour

1 cup soy flour

4 1/2 cups graham flour

● Soften yeast in 1/4 cup lukewarm water; then allow to stand for 5 minutes. Stir in honey. Combine the 2 cups water, brown-sugar replacement, oil, salt, all-purpose flour, and soy flour in a large mixing bowl. Beat to blend. Gradually beat in graham flour. Turn out onto lightly floured surface. Knead in any remaining flour. Cover and allow to rise until doubled in size. Knead slightly. Allow to rest for 5 minutes. Then form into two loaves. Place in lightly oiled loaf pans. Cover and allow to rise until doubled in size. Bake at 400°F for 50 minutes or until done.

EACH SERVING: ABOUT 98 CALORIES, 4 G PROTEIN, 18 G CARBOHYDRATE, 1 G TOTAL FAT (TRACE SATURATED), 0 MG CHOLESTEROL, 155 MG SODIUM. EXCHANGE, EACH SERVING: 1 STARCH/BREAD

PREP TIME: 15 MINUTES   COOK TIME: 35 TO 40 MINUTES
(LET RISE 2 HOURS)

Chocolate Bread

MAKES 14 SERVINGS

This chocolate-flavored yeast bread will melt in your mouth.

1 envelope dry yeast

1 cup warm water

2 1/2 cups all-purpose flour

1/2 cup unsweetened cocoa

1/2 cup granulated sugar replacement

1/2 teaspoon salt

● Sprinkle yeast over warm water in bowl. Stir and then allow to soften for 5 minutes. Combine remaining ingredients in food processor with steel blade. Process on high to blend. With food processor running, pour yeast mixture through the feeder tube. Dough will ball up and clean sides of processor bowl. Allow to process for 30 to 40 seconds. Then transfer dough to bowl or flat surface. Cover the dough loosely with plastic wrap. Allow dough to rise until double in size. Lightly oil (or spray with vegetable oil) a loaf pan. Knead dough (dough will be slightly sticky) for about 10 minutes. Form into a loaf; then place in loaf pan. Do not cover. Place in warm draft-free area until doubled in size. Bake at 400°F for 35 to 40 minutes or until done.

EACH SERVING: ABOUT 91 CALORIES, 3 G PROTEIN, 19 G CARBOHYDRATE, 1 G TOTAL FAT (TRACE SATURATED), 0 MG CHOLESTEROL, 84 MG SODIUM. EXCHANGE, EACH SERVING: 1 STARCH/BREAD

Amaretto Tea Bread

MAKES 16 SERVINGS

2 bags amaretto tea

1 cup boiling water

1 envelope dry yeast

3 1/4 cups all-purpose flour

1 tablespoon vegetable oil

1 teaspoon salt

1 teaspoon granulated sugar

● Allow tea bags to steep in the boiling water until the tea becomes very dark and lukewarm. Sprinkle yeast over tea. Stir and then allow to soften for 5 minutes. Combine flour, oil, salt, and sugar in a food processor with a steel blade. With food processor running, pour tea mixture through the feeder tube. Dough will ball up and clean sides of processor bowl. Allow to process for 30 to 40 seconds. Then transfer dough to bowl or flat surface. Cover loosely with plastic wrap. Allow dough to rise until double in size. Lightly oil (or spray with vegetable oil) a loaf pan. Knead dough (dough will be slightly sticky) for about 10 minutes. Form into a loaf; then place in loaf pan. Do not cover. Place in warm draft-free area until doubled in size. Bake at 400°F for 35 to 40 minutes or until done. Since breads made in the food processor are heavier but very flavorful, they should be cut into very thin slices.

**EACH SERVING: ABOUT 104 CALORIES, 3 G PROTEIN, 20 G CARBOHYDRATE,
1 G TOTAL FAT (TRACE SATURATED), 0 MG CHOLESTEROL, 146 MG SODIUM.
EXCHANGE, EACH SERVING: 1 STARCH/BREAD**

Quick French Bread

MAKES 24 SERVINGS

1 envelope yeast

1 1/4 cups warm water

1 teaspoon granulated sugar

1 teaspoon salt

1 tablespoon vegetable oil

3 1/4 cups all-purpose flour

● Sprinkle yeast over warm water in a large mixing bowl. Stir to blend. Allow to rest for 5 minutes. Add sugar, salt, oil, and half the flour. Beat until smooth with an electric mixer. Stir in remaining flour. Cover the bowl with plastic wrap. Allow to rise until doubled in size. Now lightly grease a cookie sheet. Form dough into an 18-inch roll. Place on cookie sheet. Do not cover. Allow to rise until doubled in size. Just before baking, brush lightly with cold water. Then bake at 350°F for 25 to 30 minutes or until done.

**EACH SERVING: ABOUT 69 CALORIES, 2 G PROTEIN, 13 G CARBOHYDRATE,
1 G TOTAL FAT (TRACE SATURATED), 0 MG CHOLESTEROL, 97 MG SODIUM.
EXCHANGE, EACH SERVING: 3/4 STARCH/BREAD**

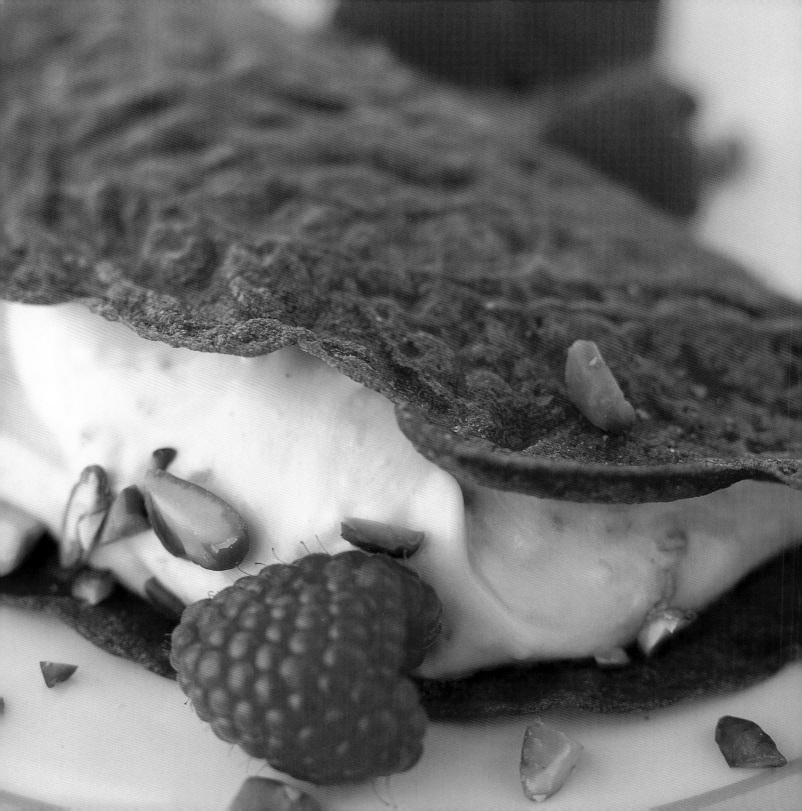

Desserts

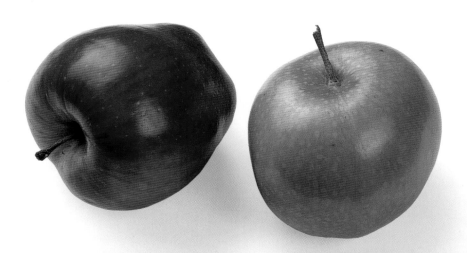

Chocolate Chocolate Mint Cake

MAKES 10 SERVINGS

1 8-ounce package sugar-free chocolate cake mix

2/3 cup water

1/2 teaspoon mint flavoring

1/2 cup mini-chocolate mint chips

2 egg whites, stiffly beaten

● Combine cake mix, water, and mint flavoring in a mixing bowl. Beat on Medium for 5 to 6 minutes or until batter is thick and creamy. Add chips. Fold in stiffly beaten egg whites. Transfer to a wax-paper-lined or greased-and-floured 8-inch round cake pan. Bake at 350°F for 20 to 25 minutes or until tester inserted in middle comes out clean. Cool in the pan for about 10 minutes; then transfer cake to rack. Cool completely.

**EACH SERVING: ABOUT 133 CALORIES
(FULL NUTRITIONAL INFORMATION NOT AVAILABLE.)
EXCHANGE, 1 SERVING: 1 BREAD, 1 1/2 FAT**

German Chocolate Cake

MAKES 3 9-INCH CAKES OR 60 SERVINGS

4 ounces baking chocolate

1/2 cup water, boiling

1/2 cup butter

1/2 cup granulated sugar replacement

3 tablespoons granulated fructose

4 egg yolks

2 teapoons vanilla extract

2 1/4 cups flour

1 teaspoon baking soda

1/2 teaspoon salt

1 cup buttermilk

4 egg whites, stiffly beaten

● Melt chocolate in boiling water; cool. Cream butter, sugar replacement, and fructose until fluffy. Add egg yolks, one at a time, beating well after each addition. Blend in vanilla and chocolate water. Sift flour with baking soda and salt; add alternately with buttermilk to chocolate mixture, beating well after each addition until smooth. Fold in beaten egg whites. Grease three 9-inch baking pans and line them with paper; grease again and lightly flour pans. Pour batter into pans. Bake at 350°F for 25 to 30 minutes or until toothpick inserted in center comes out clean. Remove from pans onto racks; remove paper lining.

**EACH SERVING: ABOUT 50 CALORIES
(FULL NUTRITIONAL INFORMATION IS NOT AVAILABLE.)
EXCHANGE, 1 SERVING: 1/2 BREAD, 1/2 FAT**

Lemon Almond Cookies

MAKES 30 COOKIES

1 8-ounce package sugar-free lemon cake mix

1 teaspoon grated lemon peel

1/2 teaspoon lemon juice

1/2 teaspoon almond flavoring

2 tablespoons water

1/4 cup slivered almonds, toasted

● Use a vegetable spray to lightly grease the cookie sheets. Combine lemon cake mix, lemon peel, lemon juice, almond flavoring, and water in a small bowl. Use a fork to completely blend. Mix in slivered almonds. Mixture will consist of large moist crumbs. Lightly dust hands with flour. Form into 30 balls. Place balls on cookie sheets. Bake at 350°F for 10 to 12 minutes. Allow cookies to cool slightly on sheets before removing.

EACH COOKIE: ABOUT 42 CALORIES, 0 G PROTEIN, 7 G CARBOHYDRATE, 2 G TOTAL FAT (TRACE SATURATED), 0 MG CHOLESTEROL, 20 MG SODIUM. EXCHANGE, 1 COOKIE: 1/3 BREAD, 1/4 FAT

Macaroon Cookies

MAKES 40 COOKIES

1 8-ounce package sugar-free white cake mix

1 egg white

1 teaspoon coconut flavoring

2 tablespoons water

3/4 cup unsweetened flaked coconut

● Use a vegetable spray to lightly grease the cookie sheets. Combine cake mix, egg white, coconut flavoring, and water in a small bowl. Beat at low speed until mixture is thoroughly blended. Blend in the flaked coconut. Drop by teaspoonfuls about 2 inches apart onto the greased cookie sheets. Bake at 375°F for 9 to 11 minutes. Allow cookies to cool slightly on sheets before removing.

EACH COOKIE: ABOUT 52 CALORIES, 0 G PROTEIN, 6 G CARBOHYDRATE, 3 G TOTAL FAT (3 G SATURATED), 0 MG CHOLESTEROL, 18 MG SODIUM. EXCHANGE, 1 COOKIE: 1/3 BREAD, 1/4 FAT

Chocolate Mousse

MAKES 10 SERVINGS

1/3 cup cocoa

1 teaspoon instant coffee

1/4 cup granulated sugar replacement

2 tablespoons cornstarch

1/4 teaspoon salt

2 cups skim milk

1 egg, beaten

8 ounces cream cheese, softened

1 teaspoon vanilla extract

● Combine cocoa, coffee, sugar replacement, cornstarch, and salt in saucepan; stir in milk. Cook and stir over medium heat until thick and bubbly; reduce heat, and then cook and stir 4 minutes longer. Remove from heat. Stir small amount of hot mixture into beaten egg and pour egg mixture into hot mixture, stirring to blend. Cook over low heat for 2 minutes and remove from heat. Add cream cheese and vanilla, beating until well blended and fluffy. Pour into 1-quart mould or dish. Cover with waxed paper and chill until firm. Remove paper and remove from mold.

**EACH SERVING: ABOUT 128 CALORIES
(FULL NUTRITIONAL INFORMATION NOT AVAILABLE.)
EXCHANGE, 1 SERVING: 1 FULL-FAT MILK, 1 FAT**

Chocolate Polka-Dot Pudding

MAKES 4 SERVINGS

1 package (4-servings) chocolate-flavored sugar-free instant pudding mix

1/4 cup mini-chocolate chips

● Make pudding mix as directed on package. Chill until set. Fold in chocolate chips. Spoon into dessert dishes.

**EACH SERVING: ABOUT 57 CALORIES, 1 G PROTEIN, 8 G CARBOHYDRATE,
3 G TOTAL FAT (2 G SATURATED), 0 MG CHOLESTEROL, 84 MG SODIUM.
EXCHANGE, 1 SERVING: 1 SKIM MILK, 1 FAT**

Chocolate Polka-Dot Pudding

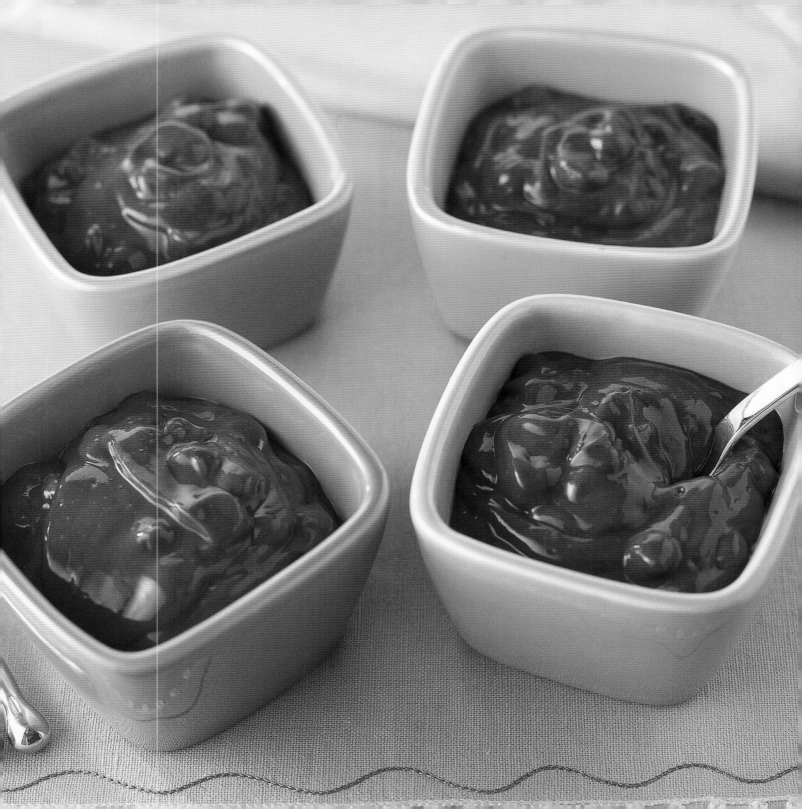

PREP TIME: 20 MINUTES   COOK TIME: 20 MINUTES

Peanut Butter Mellow Bars

MAKES 24 BARS

BASE

1 8-ounce package sugar-free white cake mix

1/4 cup chunky peanut butter

2 teaspoons water

TOPPING

2 egg whites

1/4 teaspoon vanilla flavoring

dash salt

1/4 teaspoon cream of tartar

2 tablespoons finely ground salted peanuts

● Use vegetable spray to grease an 8-inch baking pan. Combine white cake mix and peanut butter in a small bowl. Use a fork to thoroughly blend. Set aside 1/4 cup of the cake mixture. Add the 2 teaspoons of water to remaining cake mixture, and blend. Press cake mixture into the bottom of the greased pan. Combine the two egg whites, vanilla flavoring, and salt in a mixing bowl. Beat into soft peaks. Add cream of tartar and continue beating until stiff. Spread onto pressed-cake mixture in the pan. To the reserved 1/4 cup of cake mixture, add ground salted peanuts. Stir to mix. Sprinkle mixture on top of beaten egg whites in pan. Bake at 350°F for 20 minutes. Cut into 24 bars. Remove from pan and cool on rack.

EACH BAR: ABOUT 56 CALORIES, 1 G PROTEIN, 8 G CARBOHYDRATE, 2 G TOTAL FAT (TRACE SATURATED), 0 MG CHOLESTEROL, 51 MG SODIUM. EXCHANGE, 1 BAR: 1/2 BREAD, 1/2 FAT

PREP TIME: 10 MINUTES   COOK TIME: 20 MINUTES

Walnut Brownies

MAKES 24 BARS

1 8-ounce package sugar-free chocolate cake mix

1 egg yolk, beaten

1 tablespoon water

1/4 teaspoon vanilla flavoring

1/3 cup chopped walnuts

● Use a vegetable spray to lightly grease an 8-inch square cake pan. Combine chocolate cake mix, egg yolk, water, and vanilla flavoring in a small bowl. Stir to completely blend. Transfer mixture to greased pan. Sprinkle with walnuts. Bake at 350°F for 17 to 20 minutes. Cut and move from pan to cooling rack.

EACH BAR: ABOUT 51 CALORIES, 1 G PROTEIN, 8 G CARBOHYDRATE, 2 G TOTAL FAT (TRACE SATURATED), 9 MG CHOLESTEROL, 25 MG SODIUM. EXCHANGE, 1 BAR: 1/3 BREAD, 1/2 FAT

Strawberry Jelly Roll

MAKES 1 JELLY ROLL (20 SLICES)

As close to the bakery as you can get! To cut jelly-roll slices, slip a piece of 18-inch sewing thread under the roll. Crisscross the string on top of the jelly roll and pull quickly and evenly. Repeat for each slice.

1 cup cake flour, sifted

1 teaspoon baking powder

3 eggs

1/4 cup sugar replacement

3 packets concentrated acesulfame-K

1/3 cup water

1 teaspoon vanilla extract

3/4 cup fruit-only raspberry, strawberry,
*   or currant jelly*

● Spray a 15" x 10" x 1" jelly-roll pan; line the bottom with wax paper; spray the paper. Sift the flour and baking powder together. With an electric mixer, beat the eggs in a medium bowl until thick and creamy and light in color. Gradually add the sugar replacement and acesulfame-K, beating constantly until the mixture is very thick. Stir in the water and vanilla. Fold in the flour mixture. Spread the batter evenly in the prepared pan.

● Bake at 375°F for 12 minutes or until the center of the cake springs back when lightly pressed with a fingertip. Loosen the cake around the edges with a knife; invert the pan onto a clean tea towel, and peel off the wax paper. Starting at the short end, roll up the cake and towel together. Place the roll, seam side down, on a wire rack and cool completely. When cool, unroll carefully. Spread evenly with jelly. To start rerolling, lift the end of the cake using the towel. Let the towel drop and, this time, just roll the cake. Place the roll, seam side down, on a serving plate.

EACH SLICE: ABOUT 78 CALORIES, 2 G PROTEIN, 16 G CARBOHYDRATE, 1 G TOTAL FAT (TRACE SATURATED), 32 MG CHOLESTEROL, 37 MG SODIUM. EXCHANGE, EACH SLICE: 1 BREAD/STARCH

Fresh Strawberry Jelly Roll

● Follow the jelly-roll recipe above. Cool the cake on a wire rack. Just before serving, unroll and spread with 1 cup of your favorite sugar-free whipped topping and 1 cup sliced strawberries. Reroll.

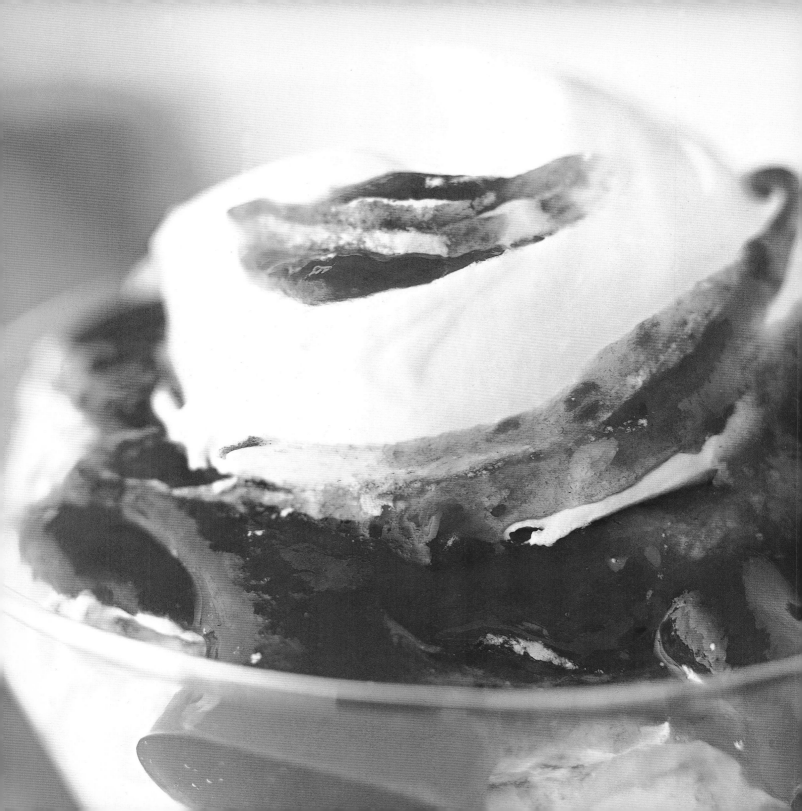

PREP TIME: 20 MINUTES

Cranberry and Raspberry Fool

MAKES 6 SERVINGS

1 1/2 cups fresh cranberries

1 1/2 cups fresh raspberries

1/4 cup granulated fructose

1/4 cup raspberry juice

2 cups prepared nondairy whipped topping

● Combine cranberries, raspberries, and fructose in a food processor or blender. Process into a purée. Transfer to a nonstick saucepan. Stir in raspberry juice. Cook and stir over medium heat until mixture is a thick purée. If desired, press through a sieve to remove seeds. Transfer mixture to a large bowl. Cover and chill mixture thoroughly. To serve: Swirl nondairy whipped topping into cranberry-raspberry mixture. Do not mix thoroughly. Divide evenly among six decorative glasses. Serve immediately.

EACH SERVING: ABOUT 69 CALORIES
(FULL NUTRITIONAL INFORMATION IS NOT AVAILABLE.)
EXCHANGE, 1 SERVING: 1/3 FRUIT, 1 FAT

PREP TIME: 10 MINUTES COOK TIME: 25 TO 30 MINUTES

Coffee Cinnamon Tart

MAKES 8 SERVINGS

2 tablespoons instant coffee powder

2 tablespoons water

3 eggs

1/4 cup granulated fructose

2 tablespoons granulated sugar replacement, measuring like sugar

1/4 teaspoon cinnamon

dash salt

9-inch unbaked tart shell, chilled

8 tablespoons prepared nondairy whipped topping

● Dissolve coffee powder in the water. Combine eggs, fructose, sugar replacement, cinnamon, and salt in a mixing bowl. Beat to blend thoroughly. Beat in coffee. Pour mixture into prepared tart shell. Bake at 350°F for 25 to 30 minutes or until middle is set. Cool completely. Just before serving, place 1 tablespoon of nondairy whipped topping on each piece.

EACH SERVING: ABOUT 166 CALORIES
(FULL NUTRITIONAL INFORMATION IS NOT AVAILABLE.)
EXCHANGE: 1 BREAD, 1 1/2 FAT

Cranberry and Raspberry Fool

PREP TIME: 25 MINUTES   COOK TIME: 25 MINUTES

Grand Marnier Soufflé for Six

MAKES 6 SERVINGS

The tricky part of soufflés is to serve them right away, when they are all puffed up.

2 *tablespoons margarine or butter*

2¹/2 *tablespoons regular all-purpose flour*

³/4 *cup skim milk*

1 *packet concentrated acesulfame-K*

2 *egg yolks, beaten*

3 *egg whites*

¹/8 *teaspoon cream of tartar*

3 *tablespoons Grand Marnier*

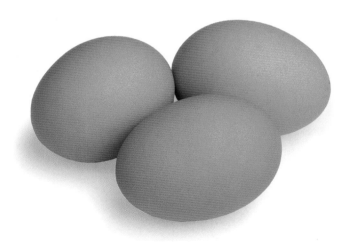

• In a saucepan, melt the margarine or butter and remove it from the heat. Stir in the flour and milk; cook, stirring over medium heat, until thickened and smooth. Stir in the acesulfame-K; cool slightly; add egg yolks.

• In a medium bowl, beat the egg whites until foamy; add the cream of tartar, beating until stiff peaks form when the beater is raised. Gently fold the egg yolk mixture and Grand Marnier into the egg whites. Turn into a one-quart soufflé dish or casserole coated with nonstick cooking spray.

• Bake for 10 minutes in a preheated 450°F oven; then turn down the heat to 325°F and bake 15 minutes longer. Serve immediately.

EACH SERVING: ABOUT 105 CALORIES, 4 G PROTEIN, 8 G CARBOHYDRATE, 6 G TOTAL FAT (1 G SATURATED), 72 MG CHOLESTEROL, 98 MG SODIUM. EXCHANGE, 1 SERVING: 1 FAT, 1 BREAD

Crisscross Peanut Butter Cookies

MAKES 60 COOKIES

1 1/2 cups all-purpose flour

1/2 teaspoon baking powder

1 cup low-sugar creamy peanut butter

1/2 cup stick margarine

2 tablespoons granulated fructose

1 large egg

1 teaspoon vanilla extract

1 cup granulated sugar replacement

● Combine flour and baking powder in a bowl. Stir to mix. Combine peanut butter, margarine, and fructose in a mixing bowl. Beat until creamy. Beat in egg, vanilla, and sweetener. Gradually add the flour mixture. (If you are using a hand mixer, you may have to stir the last part of the flour into the cookie dough.) Roll teaspoons of dough into balls. Place on ungreased cookie sheets. Flatten with a fork in a crisscross design. Bake at 375°F for 10 to 12 minutes or until cookies are golden brown. Cool slightly on cookie sheet. Then move to cooling rack.

EACH COOKIE: ABOUT 62 CALORIES
(FULL NUTRITIONAL INFORMATION IS UNAVAILABLE.)
EXCHANGE, 1 COOKIE: 1/5 BREAD, 1 FAT

Tropical Banana Pops

MAKES 6 SERVINGS

4 small bananas, crushed

1 teaspoon lemon juice

1 1/4 cups tropical sugar-free drink, from powder

1 teaspoon coconut extract or flavoring

● Put the crushed bananas into a medium bowl. Sprinkle with lemon juice and toss. Mix in the other ingredients. Spoon into six 4-ounce paper cups. Freeze until firm. To serve, peel back the paper.

EACH SERVING: ABOUT 163 CALORIES, 1 G PROTEIN, 22 G CARBOHYDRATE, 1 G TOTAL FAT (TRACE SATURATED), 0 MG CHOLESTEROL, 1,219 MG SODIUM. EXCHANGE: 1 FRUIT

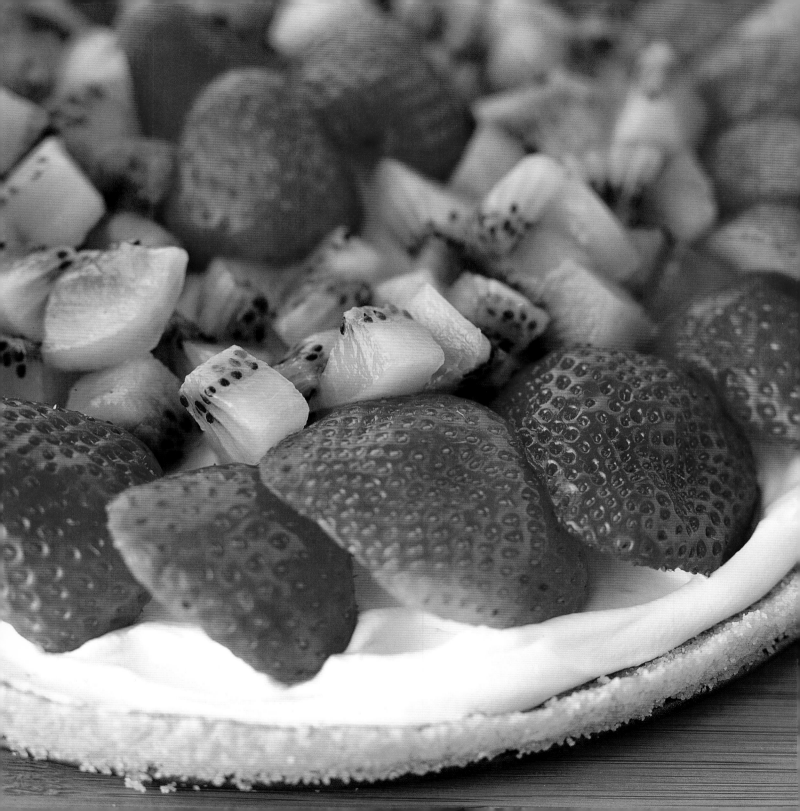

PREP TIME: 25 MINUTES

Strawberry Kiwi Torte

MAKES 10 SERVINGS

1 cup vanilla wafer crumbs

3 tablespoons melted margarine

2 cups prepared nondairy whipped topping

1 quart fresh strawberries, cleaned and sliced*

4 kiwis, cleaned and sliced

● Combine wafer crumbs and melted margarine in a bowl. Using a fork, stir to blend. Press mixture into the bottom and sides of an 8-inch lightly greased round pan to form a crust. Place in freezer to chill. Shortly before serving, spread a thick layer of nondairy whipped topping on the bottom of the crust. Place about half the strawberry slices on top of the layer of whipped topping. Spread the remaining whipped topping over the strawberries. Decorate the top of the torte with the remaining strawberry and kiwi slices. Refrigerate.

*If desired, reserve a few of the strawberries whole for extra garnish around the plate.

EACH SERVING: ABOUT 199 CALORIES, 2 G PROTEIN, 26 G CARBOHYDRATE, 10 G TOTAL FAT (3 G SATURATED), 7 MG CHOLESTEROL, 130 MG SODIUM. EXCHANGE, 1 SERVING: 1/2 BREAD, 1/2 FRUIT, 1 FAT

PREP TIME: 30 MINUTES   COOK TIME: 15 TO 20 MINUTES
(CHILL 20 MINUTES)

Quick Baked Apple Turnovers

MAKES 9 SERVINGS

1 sheet unbaked puff pastry

1 16-ounce can unsweetened sliced apples

2 teaspoons granulated fructose

1 teaspoon ground cinnamon

1 egg yolk, slightly beaten

2 tablespoons sugar-free white frosting mix

● Remove one sheet of puff pastry from carton. Allow to soften for 20 minutes; then unfold onto a lightly floured surface. Lightly flour top surface and roll into a 12-inch square. Cut into nine 4-inch squares. Slightly drain apples. Pour into a bowl; then add fructose and cinnamon. Stir or flip to coat the apple slices. Place a spoonful of apple slices in the middle of each 4" x 4" square. Lightly brush the edges of two sides of each square with the egg yolk. Fold over edges without egg yolk to seal on egg yolk edges. Place on water-sprayed cookie sheet. Chill for at least 20 minutes. Bake at 400°F for 15 to 20 minutes or until golden brown. Allow to cool. Combine frosting mix and very small amount of water in a bowl. Stir until smooth. Drizzle over top of turnovers.

EACH SERVING: ABOUT 136 CALORIES, 3 G PROTEIN, 20 G CARBOHYDRATE, 5 G TOTAL FAT (1 G SATURATED), 24 MG CHOLESTEROL, 22 MG SODIUM. EXCHANGE, 1 SERVING: 1 BREAD, 2/3 FRUIT, 1 FAT

Strawberry Kiwi Torte

Butterscotch Bars

MAKES 16 BARS

1/4 cup margarine

2/3 cup granulated brown-sugar replacement

1/3 cup granulated fructose

1 egg

1 teaspoon vanilla extract

1 cup all-purpose flour

1/4 cup chopped pecans

● Melt margarine over low heat in a medium saucepan. Remove from heat, and stir in brown-sugar replacement and fructose. Stir in egg and vanilla extract until well blended. Add flour and pecans. Stir until thoroughly blended. Spread batter evenly over the bottom of a greased 8-inch baking pan. Bake at 375°F for 20 to 25 minutes, or until golden brown. Allow to cool in pan. Cut into 16 bars.

EACH BAR: ABOUT 72 CALORIES
(FULL NUTRITIONAL INFORMATION NOT AVAILABLE.)
EXCHANGE, 1 BAR: 1/2 BREAD, 3/4 FAT

Apple Oatmeal Cookies

MAKES 36 COOKIES

1 cup all-purpose flour

1 teaspoon apple-pie spice

1/2 teaspoon baking soda

1/4 teaspoon salt

1/2 cup margarine

1/3 cup granulated sugar replacement

2 tablespoons granulated fructose

1/4 cup water

1 cup quick-cooking oatmeal

1/3 cup unsweetened dried apple slices, chopped

● Sift together flour, apple-pie spice, baking soda, and salt; set aside. Beat margarine, sugar replacement, and fructose until mixture is light and fluffy. Add water and beat well. Gradually add flour mixture to creamed mixture. Stir to blend completely. Stir in oatmeal and dried apple. Divide dough in half. Roll out dough on a floured surface to a scant 1/4-inch thickness. Cut into 18 forms, using a floured 2-inch cutter. Place on a greased cookie sheet. Roll out remaining dough and repeat cutting. Bake at 350°F for 10 minutes, or until lightly browned. Move to cooling rack.

EACH COOKIE: ABOUT 63 CALORIES, 1 G PROTEIN, 8 G CARBOHYDRATE,
3 G TOTAL FAT (1 G SATURATED), 0 MG CHOLESTEROL, 86 MG SODIUM.
EXCHANGE, 1 COOKIE: 1/3 BREAD

PREP TIME: 25 MINUTES   COOK TIME: 40 MINUTES

Granola Cheesecake

MAKES 10 SERVINGS

A super combination—creamy cheesecake with a crunch.

CRUST

1/4 cup margarine or butter, melted

1 tablespoon water

3 packets concentrated acesulfame-K

1 cup Granola Topping (recipe follows)

FILLING

8 ounces nonfat cream cheese, softened

1 cup nonfat cottage cheese, drained

1/2 cup egg substitute or 2 eggs

3 packets concentrated acesulfame-K

1 teaspoon vanilla extract

1 tablespoon flour

TOPPING

1/3 cup Granola Topping (recipe follows)

● Stir the crust ingredients together and press the mixture into the bottom of a greased and floured 9-inch springform pan. Set aside. Beat the filling ingredients together until smooth. Spoon this carefully over the crust. Sprinkle the top with granola topping. Bake in a 375°F oven for 40 minutes or until set. Cool before removing cake from the pan.

EACH SERVING (WITHOUT TOPPING): ABOUT 150 CALORIES, 9 G PROTEIN, 4 G CARBOHYDRATE, 11 G TOTAL FAT (2 G SATURATED), 45 MG CHOLESTEROL, 202 MG SODIUM. EXCHANGE, 1 SERVING: 1 MEAT

Granola Topping

MAKES 4 1/2 CUPS

3 cups oatmeal

1/2 cup wheat germ

2/3 cup sliced almonds (optional)

1 tablespoon safflower oil

2 tablespoons molasses

1/2 cup unsweetened apple juice

● Mix the oatmeal, wheat germ, and almonds, if using, in a lasagna or jelly-roll pan. Heat the remaining ingredients in a saucepan and stir to combine. Drizzle this over the oatmeal mixture; then use a spatula to push the mixture around in the pan until it is evenly coated. Bake in a 325°F oven for about 30 minutes. Then mix again and bake for 10 minutes. The longer you cook it, the crunchier the granola gets.

EACH TABLESPOON: ABOUT 27 CALORIES, 1 G PROTEIN, 3 G CARBOHYDRATE, 1 G TOTAL FAT (0 G SATURATED), 0 MG CHOLESTEROL, 34 MG SODIUM. EXCHANGE: NEGLIGIBLE

Chocolate Crêpes with Pistachio Cream and Raspberries

MAKES 8 SERVINGS

1 package (4 servings) sugar-free instant pistachio
*   pudding mix*
1 egg white
1/2 cup prepared nondairy whipped topping
8 Chocolate Crêpes (recipe follows)
32 fresh ripe raspberries

● Prepare pistachio pudding mix as directed on package. Set until firm. Beat egg white until stiff. Fold a small amount of egg white into pistachio pudding to loosen. Fold pudding into egg white. Carefully fold in nondairy whipped topping. To assemble: Place crepes on dessert plates. Fill one-half of each crepe with pistachio filling. Fold crepes in half, covering the pistachio filling. Lay four raspberries next to each crepe.

EACH SERVING: ABOUT 66 CALORIES, 3 G PROTEIN, 8 G CARBOHYDRATE, 3 G TOTAL FAT (1 G SATURATED), 29 MG CHOLESTEROL, 84 MG SODIUM. EXCHANGE, 1 SERVING: 1 BREAD

Chocolate Crêpes

MAKES 8 SERVINGS

1/4 cup skim milk
6 tablespoons all-purpose flour
2 tablespoons unsweetened cocoa powder
dash salt
1 teaspoon granulated fructose
1 egg
2 teaspoons vegetable oil

● Combine all ingredients in order given in a blender or bowl. Beat until blended and smooth. Cover and refrigerate 1 to 24 hours. To fry: Batter should be the consistency of light cream. If necessary, add a small amount of water to batter. Heat an 8-inch nonstick skillet or crêpe iron over medium heat until a drop of water sizzles when sprinkled on the surface. Reduce heat a little. Use crêpe iron as directed by manufacturer. Spray nonstick skillet with a vegetable-oil spray. Remove skillet from heat. Spoon in 2 tablespoons of batter. Tilt skillet in a circle to spread batter around bottom. Return to heat, and brown crêpe on one side. Invert pan over a plate or paper towel. Repeat using remaining batter.

EACH SERVING: ABOUT 49 CALORIES, 2 G PROTEIN, 6 G CARBOHYDRATE, 2 G TOTAL FAT (1 G SATURATED), 27 MG CHOLESTEROL, 32 MG SODIUM. EXCHANGE, 1 CRÊPE: 2/3 BREAD

Chocolate Crêpes with Pistachio Cream and Raspberries

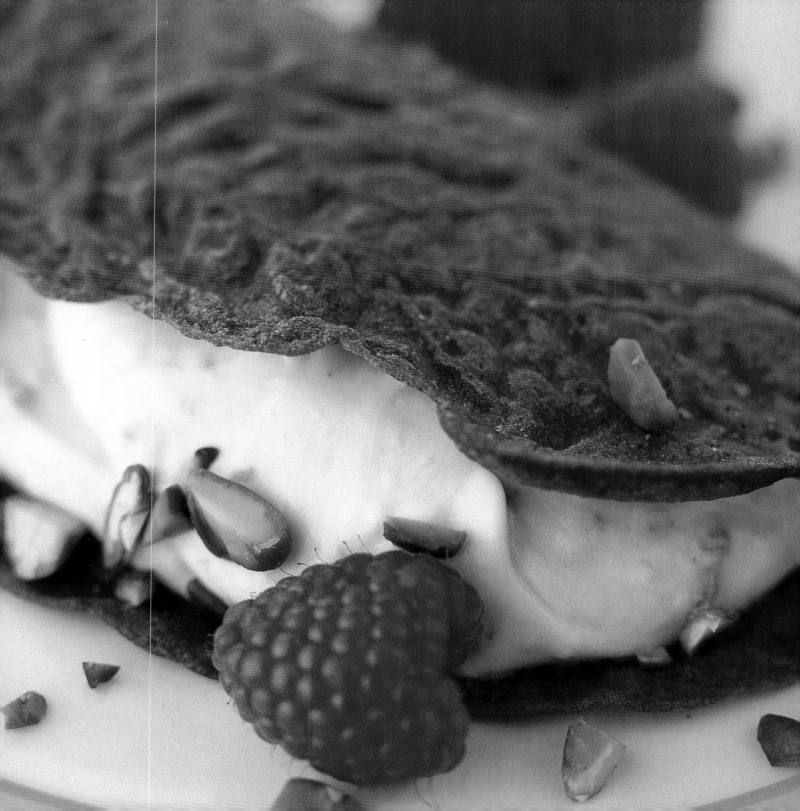

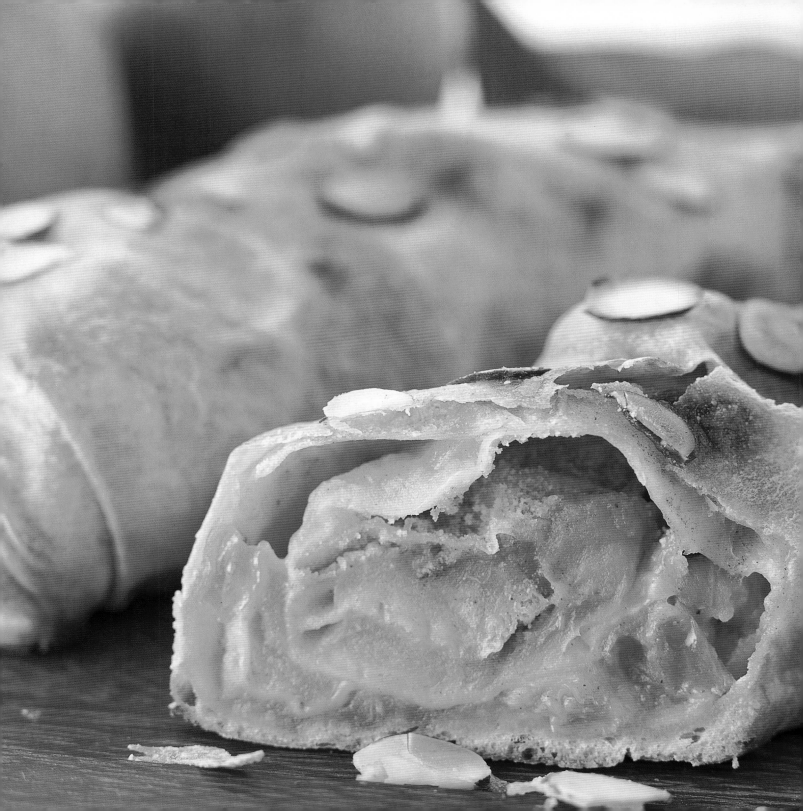

German Apple Strudel

MAKES 16 SLICES

Apple strudel oozes good feelings and a hearty welcome. Your family and guests will be very impressed.

DOUGH

2 cups flour

1 large egg or equivalent egg substitute, lightly beaten

1 tablespoon canola oil

1/2 teaspoon salt

2/3 cup warm water

FILLING

4 tablespoons butter, margarine, or fat-free butter and oil replacement

1/2 cup dry bread crumbs

4 large apples, peeled, cored, and sliced

1/4 cup sugar

1 tablespoon cinnamon

1/2 cup raisins

GLAZE FROSTING

1 large egg yolk

1 teaspoon sugar

1 tablespoon water

● Put the flour in a mixing bowl. In another bowl, mix together the egg, oil, salt, and warm water. Pour the liquid onto the flour and mix thoroughly. Turn out onto a well-floured work surface. Knead the dough until it is smooth and elastic. Cover with a tea towel or plastic wrap and let sit for 15 minutes. Meanwhile, make the filling by melting the butter in a saucepan. Add the bread crumbs and brown just until golden. Roll out the dough on a well-floured work surface. Make it as thin as possible. Sprinkle the bread crumbs evenly over the surface of the dough. In a mixing bowl, coat the apple slices with the sugar and cinnamon by tossing lightly. Add the raisins and mix again. Spread this mixture evenly on top of the bread crumbs. Roll up the long way. Seal the dough together with your fingers. Mix the egg yolk, half the sugar, and water together and brush the top of the roll. Sprinkle the top with remaining sugar. Bake in a preheated 400°F oven for 30 to 35 minutes. Serve hot or cold.

EACH SERVING: ABOUT 165 CALORIES, 3 G PROTEIN, 28 G CARBOHYDRATE, 5 G TOTAL FAT (2 G SATURATED), 34 MG CHOLESTEROL, 136 MG SODIUM. EXCHANGE, EACH SLICE: 1 STARCH, 1/2 FRUIT, 1 FAT

Italian Fig Cookies

MAKES 24 LARGE COOKIES

The little "figlets" are fine in this recipe, too; just be sure they aren't sweetened.

1 1/2 *cups figs, dried*

3/4 *cup raisins*

1/4 *cup almonds, slivered*

1/4 *cup and 2 tablespoons sugar*

1/4 *cup hot water*

1/4 *teaspoon ground cinnamon*

1 *dash pepper*

2 1/2 *cups all-purpose flour*

1/4 *teaspoon baking powder*

10 *tablespoons butter, margarine, or fat-free butter and oil replacement*

1/2 *cup lowfat 1% milk*

1 *large egg or equivalent egg substitute, beaten*

● Chop figs, raisins, and almonds together in a food processor. In a mixing bowl, combine the 2 tablespoons sugar , hot water, cinnamon, and pepper. Add the chopped-fruit mixture. Set aside. In another mixing bowl, combine the flour, 1/4 cup sugar, and baking powder. Cut in the butter, and blend until the pieces are the size of small peas. Stir in the milk and egg until all the dry mixture is moistened. Divide the dough in half. On a lightly floured work surface, roll each half into an 18" x 16" rectangle. Cut each rectangle into four 18" x 4" strips. Spread about 1/3 cup of the fig mixture over each strip of dough. Roll the dough up jelly-roll fashion, starting at the long side. Cut each filled strip into six 3-inch lengths. Place the cookies, seam side down, on ungreased cookie sheets. Curve each cookie slightly. Snip the outer edge of the curve three times. Bake in a preheated 350°F oven until lightly browned, 20 to 25 minutes. Remove from cookie sheets and cool on a rack.

EACH SERVING: ABOUT 130 CALORIES, 2 G PROTEIN, 17 G CARBOHYDRATE, 6 G TOTAL FAT (3 G SATURATED), 22 MG CHOLESTEROL, 61 MG SODIUM. EXCHANGE, EACH COOKIE: 1 STARCH, 1 FRUIT, 1/2 FAT

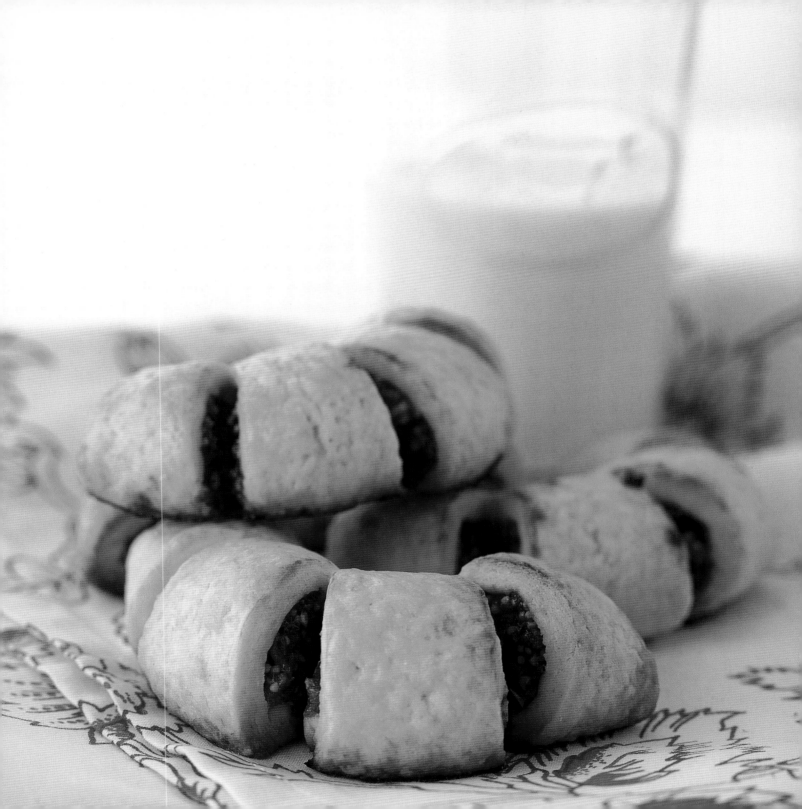

Pavlova Wedges with Kiwis and Raspberry Sauce

MAKES 8 SERVINGS

1 recipe Basic Meringue (page 207)
4 ripe kiwis
1 recipe Raspberry Sauce (recipe follows)

● Prepare the Basic Meringue. Trace a 12-inch circle on the inside of a clean brown paper grocery bag or a piece of parchment paper. Put the paper on an ungreased cookie sheet. Spoon the meringue into the circle. Spread the meringue so it is evenly distributed. Bake in a preheated 250°F oven for 1 hour. Turn off the oven. Leave the meringue in the oven for an additional 30 minutes without opening the door. Carefully cut the meringue into eight wedges. Put each wedge on a dessert plate. Peel the kiwis. Slice thinly. Arrange one-half sliced kiwi on each slice of meringue. Spoon raspberry sauce over the fruit and meringue.

EACH SERVING: ABOUT 125 CALORIES, 2 G PROTEIN, 28 G CARBOHYDRATE,
TRACE TOTAL FAT (0 G SATURATED), 0 MG CHOLESTEROL, 29 MG SODIUM.
EXCHANGE, EACH SERVING: 1 STARCH/BREAD, 1/2 FRUIT

Raspberry Sauce

MAKES 3/4 CUP (8 SERVINGS)

1/2 cup no-sugar-added seedless raspberry preserves
2 tablespoons Chambord liqueur or raspberry brandy
2 tablespoons water

● Put the preserves into a small saucepan. Add the raspberry liqueur and water. Mix well with a wire whisk. Heat gently, stirring constantly.

EACH SERVING: ABOUT 71 CALORIES, 0 G PROTEIN, 16 G CARBOHYDRATE,
0 G TOTAL FAT (0 G SATURATED), 0 MG CHOLESTEROL, 7 MG SODIUM.
EXCHANGE, EACH SERVING: 1/2 FRUIT

PREP TIME: 20 MINUTES   COOK TIME: 3 HOURS

Basic Meringue

MAKES 4 SERVINGS

3 *large egg whites*

1/4 teaspoon cream of tartar

1/4 cup sugar

● Preheat the over to 250°F or the temperature specified in the specific recipe. Cut a brown paper grocery bag or parchment paper to the same size as your cookie sheet. Place the paper on top of the cookie sheet. Using plates, cups, or saucers and a pencil, trace the shape specified in the recipe onto the paper. In a large glass or metal bowl, beat the egg whites with the cream of tartar using an electric mixer. When soft peaks begin to form, keep beating, but slowly add the sugar. Increase the mixer speed until stiff peaks form and the meringue is glossy. Don't beat past this point or the meringue will become too dry!

● With a clean spoon or rubber scraper, transfer the beaten egg white to the circles drawn on the paper. Bake in a 250°F preheated oven for the amount of time specified in the recipe. When the time is up, turn off the oven but don't open the oven door. Leave the meringues in the cooling oven for 2 more hours. Then carefully remove the cookie sheets from the oven. Use a spatula to loosen the meringue from the paper.

EACH SERVING: ABOUT 61 CALORIES, 3 G PROTEIN, 13 G CARBOHYDRATE, 0 G TOTAL FAT (0 G SATURATED), 0 MG CHOLESTEROL, 41 MG SODIUM. EXCHANGE, EACH SERVING: 1 STARCH/BREAD

PREP TIME: 15 MINUTES (FREEZE 2 TO 3 HOURS)

Strawberry Ice Cream Pie

MAKES 8 SERVINGS

Let the ice cream soften before beginning the rest of the recipe.

1 packet (4 servings) sugar-free strawberry gelatin powder

2/3 cup boiling water

2 cups sugar-free low-fat strawberry ice cream, softened

1 cup frozen low-fat nondairy whipped topping, thawed

1 frozen pie crust, baked

1 cup fresh or frozen (no sugar added) strawberries (optional)

● Put the gelatin powder into a large mixing bowl. Add the boiling water. Stir until gelatin is dissolved. Add the ice cream slowly. Stir until the mixture is smooth (except for the strawberry pieces, of course). Stir in the whipped topping by spoonfuls. Beat after each addition (a whisk works well). Spoon the mixture into the prepared pie crust. Freeze a few hours until firm. For easiest cutting, run a sharp knife under hot running water between each cut. Garnish with strawberries and whipped topping, if desired.

EACH SERVING: ABOUT 128 CALORIES (FULL NUTRITIONAL INFORMATION UNAVAILABLE.) EXCHANGE, EACH SERVING: 1 STARCH/BREAD; 1 FAT

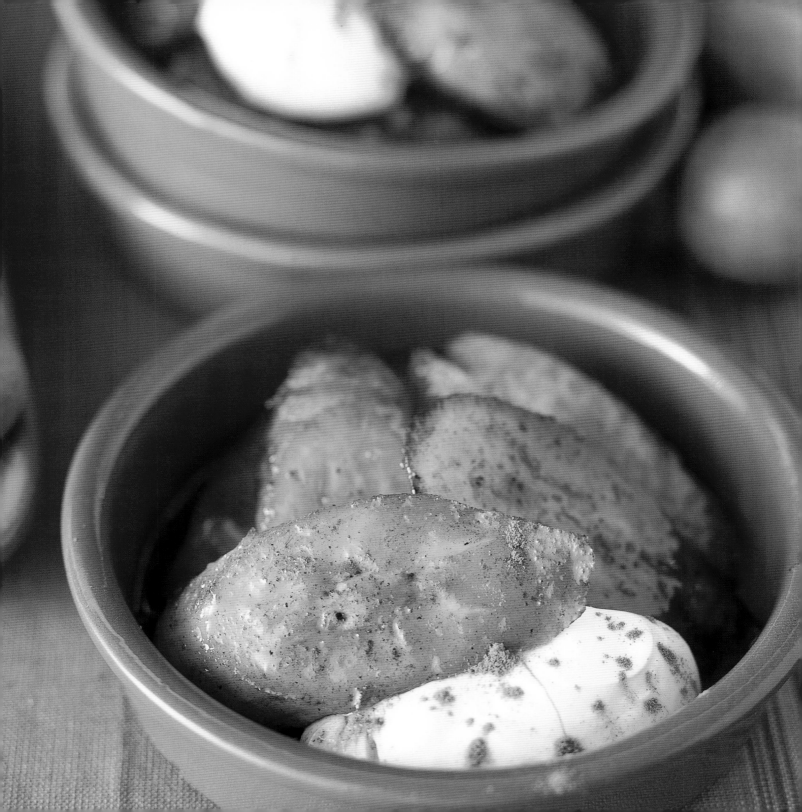

Brown Sugar Plantains and Cream

MAKES 4 SERVINGS

I always look for these on menus in Cuban restaurants. Use bananas if you can't get plantains.

3 *tablespoons butter or margarine*

2 *tablespoons brown sugar*

1 *teaspoon vanilla*

1/4 *teaspoon cinnamon*

2 *cups sliced plantains or bananas*

1/4 *cup low-fat frozen nondairy whipped topping*

2 *tablespoons toasted slivered almonds*

• Melt the butter over low heat in a large skillet. Add the brown sugar, vanilla, and cinnamon. Stir. Add the plantains and stir gently to coat. Remove from heat. Spoon into four serving bowls. Top with whipped topping and almonds.

EACH SERVING: ABOUT 200 CALORIES, 2 G PROTEIN, 24 G CARBOHYDRATE, 12 G TOTAL FAT (6 G SATURATED), 26 MG CHOLESTEROL, 96 MG SODIUM. EXCHANGE, EACH SERVING: 2 STARCH, 1 FAT

Chocolate Drizzle

MAKES 1/3 CUP

This is great drizzled over chocolate cake—for an extra special treat, make the German Chocolate Cake (page 186), spread Chocolate Mousse (page 188) between layers, and top with Chocolate Drizzle.

2 *teaspoons cornstarch*

1/4 *cup cold water*

dash salt

1 *ounce baking chocolate*

1/3 *cup granulated sugar replacement*

1/2 *teaspoon butter*

• Blend cornstarch and cold water and pour into a small saucepan. Add salt and chocolate. Cook on low heat until chocolate melts and mixture is thick; remove from heat. Stir in sugar replacement and blend in butter. Use over cake or ice cream.

CALORIES: NEGLIGIBLE, EXCHANGE: NEGLIGIBLE

Brown Sugar Plantains and Cream

Italian Rice Pudding Torte

MAKES 12 SERVINGS

Drier than northern European rice puddings, this is more like a cake. It's delicious with fancy coffee.

4 cups water

1/2 cup rice

7 large eggs or equivalent egg substitute

1/2 cup sugar

1/4 cup rum

4 teaspoons grated lemon or lime peel

2 tablespoons grated orange peel

2 teaspoons vanilla extract

1/4 teaspoon salt

2 tablespoons lowfat 1% milk

● Combine the water and rice in a heavy saucepan and cook over medium heat until boiling. Lower heat and let simmer for 10 minutes. Drain the rice and let it cool. In an electric mixing bowl, beat the eggs well. Add the sugar and continue beating until very pale. Add the rum, lemon or lime peel, orange peel, vanilla extract, and salt. Mix well. Whisk in the milk.

● Butter a 9-inch round baking dish. Spread the rice on the bottom and pour the milk mixture over it. Bake in a preheated 350°F oven for about 45 minutes, until the top is a deep golden color.

EACH SERVING: ABOUT 128 CALORIES, 6 G PROTEIN, 14 G CARBOHYDRATE, 4 G TOTAL FAT (1 G SATURATED), 126 MG CHOLESTEROL, 123 MG SODIUM. EXCHANGE, EACH SERVING: 1 LOWFAT MILK

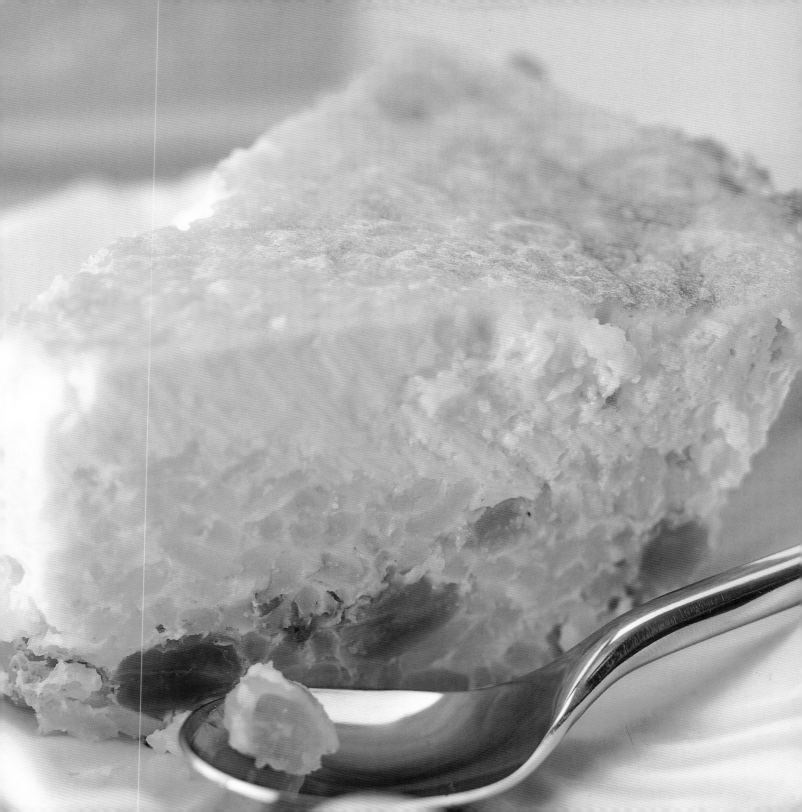

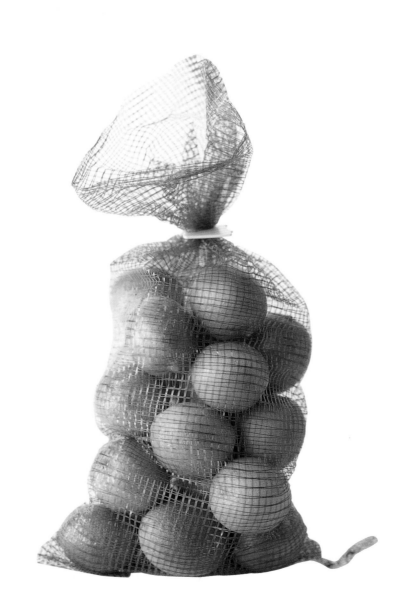

Food Exchange Lists

	Carbohydrate (grams)	Protein (grams)	Fat (grams)	Calories (grams)
I. Starch/bread	15	3	trace	80
II. Meat				
Very lean	—	7	0–1	35
Lean	—	7	3	55
Medium-fat	—	7	5	75
High-fat	—	7	8	100
III. Vegetable	5	2	—	25
IV. Fruit	15	—	—	60
V. Milk				
Skim	12	8	0–3	90
Low-fat	12	8	5	120
Whole	12	8	8	150
VI. Fat	—	—	5	45

CEREALS/GRAINS/PASTA

1/2 cup of cereal, grain, or pasta = one serving

Bran cereals, concentrated (such as Bran Buds, All Bran)†	1/3 cup
Bran cereals, flaked†	1/2 cup
Bulgur (cooked)	1/2 cup
Cooked cereals	1/2 cup
Cornmeal (dry)	2 1/2 tbsp
Grape Nuts	3 tbsp
Grits (cooked)	1/2 cup
Other ready-to-eat, unsweetened (plain) cereals	3/4 cup
Pasta (cooked)	1/2 cup
Puffed cereal	1 1/2 cups
Rice, white or brown (cooked)	1/3 cup
Shredded wheat	1/2 cup
Wheat germ†	3 tbsp

DRIED BEANS/PEAS/LENTILS

Beans and peas (cooked) (such as kidney, white, split, blackeye)†	1/3 cup
Lentils (cooked)†	1/3 cup
Baked beans†	1/4 cup

STARCHY VEGETABLES

Corn†	1/2 cup
Corn on the cob, 6 in.†	1 long
Lima beans†	1/2 cup
Peas, green (canned or frozen)†	1/2 cup
Plaintain†	1/2 cup
Potato, baked, 1 small	3 oz
Potato, mashed	1/2 cup
Squash, winter (acorn, butternut)	3/4 cup
Yam, sweet potato	1/3 cup

BREAD

Bagel	1/2 (1 oz)
Bread sticks, crisp, 4 in. long x 1/2 in.	2 (2/3 oz)
Croutons low fat	1 cup
English muffin	1/2
Frankfurter or hamburger bun	1/2 (1 oz)
Pita, 6 in. diameter	1/2
Plain roll, small	1 (1 oz)
Raisin, unfrosted	1 slice
Rye, pumpernickel†	1 slice (1 oz)
Tortilla, 6 in. diameter	1
White (including French, Italian)	1 slice (1 oz)
Whole wheat	1 slice

† = 3 grams or more of fiber per serving.

CRACKERS/SNACKS

Animal crackers	8
Graham crackers, $2^1/2$ in. square	3
Matzoh	$3/4$ oz
Melba toast	5 slices
Oyster crackers	24
Popcorn (popped, no fat added)	3 cups
Pretzels	$3/4$ oz
Rye crisps (2 in. x $3^1/2$ in.)	4
Saltine-type crackers	6
Whole-wheat crackers, no fat added (crisp breads such as Finn, Kavli, Wasa)	2–4 slices ($3/4$ oz)

STARCHY FOODS PREPARED WITH FAT
(count as 1 starch/bread serving, plus 1 fat serving)

Biscuit, $2^1/2$ in. across	1
Chow mein noodles	$1/2$ cup
Corn bread, 2-in. cube	1 (2 oz)
Cracker, round butter type	6
French-fried potatoes (2 in. to $3^1/2$ in. long)	10 ($1^1/2$ oz)
Muffin, plain, small	1
Pancake, 4 in. diameter	2
Stuffing, bread (prepared)	$1/4$ cup
Taco shell, 6 in. diameter	2
Waffle, $4^1/2$ in. square	1
Whole-wheat crackers, fat added (such as Triscuits)	4–6 (1 oz)

II. Meat List

	Carbohydrate (grams)	Protein (grams)	Fat (grams)	Calories
Very lean	0	7	0–1	35
Lean	0	7	3	55
Medium-fat	0	7	5	75
High-fat	0	7	8	100

‡ = 400 mg or more of sodium per serving.

Lean Meat and Substitutes
One exchange is equal to any one of the following items:

Beef	USDA Good or Choice grade of lean beef, such as round, sirloin, and flank steak; tenderloin; and chipped beef ‡	1 oz
Pork	Lean pork, such as fresh ham; canned, cured, or boiled ham‡, Canadian bacon‡, tenderloin	1 oz
Veal	All cuts are lean except for veal cutlets (ground or cubed)	1 oz
Poultry	Chicken, turkey, Cornish hen (without skin)	1 oz
Fish	All fresh and frozen fish	1 oz
	Crab, lobster, scallops, shrimp, clams (fresh, or canned in water‡)	2 oz
	Oysters	6 med
	Tuna (canned in water)‡	$1/4$ cup
	Herring (uncreamed or smoked)	1 oz
	Sardines (canned)	2 med
Wild Game	Venison, rabbit, squirrel	1 oz
	Pheasant, duck, goose (without skin)	1 oz
Cheese	Any cottage cheese	$1/4$ cup
	Grated Parmesan	2 tbsp
	Diet cheese‡ (with fewer than 55 calories per ounce)	1 oz
Other	95% fat-free luncheon meat	1 oz
	Egg whites	3
	Egg substitutes (with fewer than 55 calories per $1/4$ cup)	$1/4$ cup

Medium-Fat and Meat Substitutes
One exchange is equal to any one of the following items:

Beef	Most beef products fall into this category. Examples: all ground beef, roast (rib, chuck, rump), steak (cubed, Porterhouse, T-bone), and meat loaf.	1 oz
Pork	Most pork products fall into this category. Examples: chops, loin roast, Boston butt, cutlets	1 oz
Lamb	Most lamb products fall into this category Examples: chops, leg, roast	1 oz
Veal	Cutlet (ground or cubed, unbreaded)	1 oz

Poultry	Chicken (with skin), domestic duck or goose (well drained of fat), ground turkey	1 oz
Fish	Tuna (canned in oil and drained)‡	1/4 cup
	Salmon (canned)‡	1/4 cup
Cheese	Skim or part-skim milk cheeses, such as:	
	Ricotta	1/4 cup
	Mozzarella	1 oz
	Diet cheeses‡ (with 56–80 calories per ounce)	1 oz
Other	86% fat-free luncheon meat‡	1 oz
	Egg (high in cholesterol, so limit to 3 per week)	1
	Egg substitutes (with 56–80 calories per 1/4 cup)	1/4 cup
	Tofu (2 1/2 in. x 2 3/4 in. x 1 in.)	4 oz
	Liver, heart, kidney, sweetbreads (high in cholesterol)	1 oz

High-Fat Meat and Substitutes

Remember, these items are high in saturated fat, cholesterol, and calories, and should be eaten only three times per week.

One exchange is equal to any one of the following items:

Beef	Most USDA Prime cuts of beef, such as ribs, corned beef‡	1 oz
Pork	Spareribs, ground pork, pork sausage (patty or link)‡	1 oz
Lamb	Patties (ground lamb)	1 oz
Fish	Any fried fish product	1 oz
Cheese	All regular cheese‡, such as American, blue, Cheddar, Monterey, Swiss	1 oz
Other	Luncheon meat‡, such as bologna, salami, pimiento loaf	1 oz
	Sausage‡, such as Polish, Italian	1 oz
	Knockwurst, smoked	1 oz
	Bratwurst‡	1 oz
	Frankfurter (turkey or chicken)‡ (10/lb)	1 frank
	Peanut butter (contains unsaturated fat)	1 tbsp

Count as one high-fat meat plus one fat exchange:

	Frankfurter (beef, pork, or combination)‡ (400 mg or more of sodium per exchange) (10/lb)	1 frank

III. Vegetable List

1/2 cup cooked vegetables or vegetable juice

1 cup raw vegetables

Artichoke (1/2 medium)

Eggplant

Asparagus

Greens (collard, mustard, turnip)

Beans (green, wax, Italian)

Kohlrabi

Bean sprouts

Leeks

Beets

Mushrooms, cooked

Broccoli

Okra

Brussels sprouts

Onions

Cabbage, cooked

Pea pods

Carrots

Peppers (green)

Cauliflower

Tomato (one large)

Rutabaga

Tomato/vegetable juice‡

Sauerkraut‡

Turnips

Spinach, cooked

Water chestnuts

Summer squash (crookneck)

Zucchini, cooked

Starchy vegetables such as corn, peas, and potatoes are found on the Starch/Bread List.

For "free" vegetables (i.e., fewer than ten calories per serving), see the Free Food List.

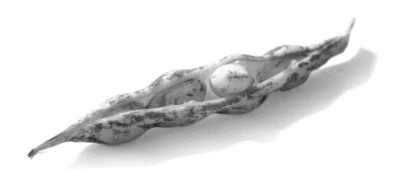

‡ = 400 mg or more of sodium per serving.

IV. Fruit List

1/2 cup of fresh fruit or fruit juice
1/4 cup dried fruit

Fresh, Frozen, and Unsweetened Canned Fruit

Apples (raw, 2 in. diameter)	1
Applesauce (unsweetened)	1/2 cup
Apricots (canned) (4 halves)	1/2 cup
Banana (9 in. long)	1/2
Blackberries (raw)	3/4 cup
Blueberries (raw)†	3/4 cup
Cantaloupe (5 in. diameter)	1/3
Cantaloupe (cubes)	1 cup
Cherries (large, raw)	12 whole
Cherries (canned)	1/2 cup
Figs (raw, 2 in. diameter)	2
Fruit cocktail (canned)	1/2 cup
Grapefruit (medium)	1/2
Grapefruit (segments)	3/4 cup
Grapes (small)	15
Honeydew melon (medium)	1/8
Honeydew melon (cubes)	1 cup
Kiwi (large)	1
Mandarin oranges	3/4 cup
Mango (small)	1/2
Nectarines (2 1/2 in. diameter)	1
Orange (2 1/2 in. diameter)	1
Papaya	1 cup
Peach (2 3/4 in. diameter)	1
Peaches (canned) (2 halves)	1 cup
Pear (1/2 large)	1 small
Pears (canned) (2 halves)	1/2 cup
Persimmon (medium, native)	2
Pineapple (raw)	3/4 cup
Pineapple (canned)	1/3 cup
Plum (raw, 2 in. diameter)	2
Pomegranate†	1/2
Raspberries (raw)†	1 cup
Strawberries (raw, whole)†	1 1/4 cups
Tangerine (2 1/2 in. diameter)	2
Watermelon (cubes)	1 1/4 cups

Dried Fruit†

Apples†	4 rings
Apricots†	7 halves
Dates (medium)	2 1/2
Figs†	1 1/2
Prunes (medium)†	3
Raisins	2 tbsp

Fruit Juice

Apple juice/cider	1/2 cup
Cranberry juice cocktail	1/3 cup
Grapefruit juice	1/2 cup
Grape juice	1/3 cup
Orange juice	1/2 cup
Pineapple juice	1/2 cup
Prune juice	1/3 cup

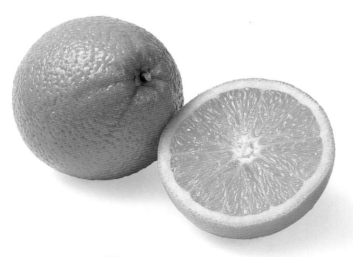

† = 3 grams or more of fiber per serving.
‡ = 400 mg or more of sodium per serving.

V. Milk List

Milk	Carbohydrate (grams)	Protein (grams)	Fat (grams)	Calories
Skim	12	8	trace	90
Low-fat	12	8	5	120
Whole	12	8	8	150

Skim and Very Low-Fat Milk

Skim milk	1 cup
1/2% milk	1 cup
1% milk	1 cup
Low-fat buttermilk	1 cup
Evaporated skim milk	1/2 cup
Dry nonfat milk	1/3 cup
Plain nonfat yogurt	8 oz.

Low-Fat Milk

2% milk	1 cup
Plain low-fat yogurt (with added nonfat milk solids)	8 oz.

Whole Milk

The whole-milk group has much more fat per serving than the skim and low-fat groups. Whole milk has more than 3 1/4% butterfat. Try to limit your choices from the whole-milk group as much as possible.

Whole milk	1 cup
Evaporated whole milk	1/2 cup
Whole-milk plain yogurt	8 oz.

VI. Fat List

Unsaturated Fats

Avocado	1/8 medium
Margarine	1 tsp
Margarine, diet‡	1 tbsp
Mayonnaise	1 tsp
Mayonnaise (reduced-calorie)‡	1 tbsp

Nuts and Seeds:

Almonds, dry roasted	6
Cashews, dry roasted	1 tbsp
Pecans	2
Peanuts (small)	20
Peanuts (large)	10
Walnuts	2 whole
Other nuts	1 tbsp
Seeds (except pumpkin), pine nuts, sunflower (without shells)	1 tbsp
Pumpkin seeds	2 tsp
Oil (corn, cottonseed, safflower, soybean, sunflower, olive, peanut)	1 tsp
Olives (small)‡	10
Olives (large)‡	5
Salad dressing, mayonnaise-type, regular	2 tsp
Salad dressing, mayonnaise-type, reduced-calorie	1 tbsp
Salad dressing, all varieties, regular	1 tbsp
Salad dressing, reduced-calorie‡ (2 tbsp of low-calorie dressing is a free food)	2 tbsp

Saturated Fats

Butter	1 tsp
Bacon‡	1 slice
Chitterlings	1/2 oz
Coconut, shredded	2 tbsp
Coffee whitener, liquid	2 tbsp
Coffee whitener, powder	4 tsp
Cream (light, coffee, table)	2 tbsp
Cream, sour	2 tbsp
Cream (heavy, whipping)	1 tbsp
Cream cheese	1 tbsp
Salt pork‡	1/4 oz

† = 3 grams or more of fiber per serving.
‡ = 400 mg or more of sodium per serving.

Free Foods

Drinks

Bouillon or broth without fat‡

Bouillon, low-sodium

Carbonated drinks, sugar-free

Carbonated water

Club soda

Cocoa powder, unsweetened (1 tbsp)

Coffee/tea

Drink mixes, sugar-free

Tonic water, sugar-free

Fruit

Cranberries, unsweetened (1/2 cup)

Rhubarb, unsweetened (1/2 cup)

Vegetables (raw, 1 cup)

Cabbage

Celery

Chinese cabbage†

Cucumber

Green onion

Hot peppers

Mushrooms

Radishes

Zucchini†

Salad Greens

Endive

Escarole

Lettuce

Romaine

Spinach

Sweets

Candy, hard, sugar-free

Gelatin, sugar-free

Gum, sugar-free

Jam/jelly, sugar-free (2 tsp)

Pancake syrup, sugar-free (1–2 tbsp)

Sugar substitutes (saccharin, aspartame)

Whipped topping (2 tbsp)

Condiments

Ketchup (1 tbsp)

Horseradish

Mustard

Pickles, dill, unsweetened‡

Salad dressing, low-calorie (2 tbsp)

Taco sauce (1 tbsp)

Vinegar

Nonstick pan spray

Seasonings

Seasonings can be very helpful in making foods taste better. Be careful of how much sodium you use. Read labels to help you choose seasonings that do not contain sodium or salt.

Basil (fresh)

Celery Seeds

Cinnamon

Chili powder

Chives

Curry

Dill

Flavoring extracts (vanilla, almond, walnut, butter, peppermint, lemon, etc.)

Garlic

Garlic powder

Herbs

Hot pepper sauce

Lemon

Lemon juice

Lemon pepper

Lime

Lime Juice

Mint

Onion powder

Oregano

Paprika

Pepper

Pimiento

Spices

Soy sauce‡

Soy sauce, low sodium (light)

Wine, used in cooking (1/4 cup)

Worcestershire sauce

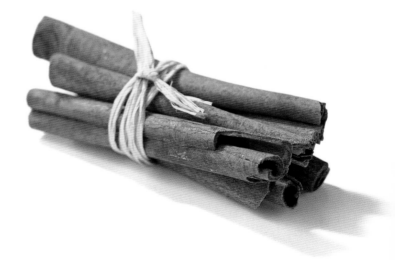

† = 3 grams or more of fiber per serving.
‡ = 400mg or more of sodium per serving.

Combination Foods

Food	Amount	Exchanges
Casserole, homemade	1 cup (8 oz)	2 medium-fat meat, 2 starches, 1 fat
Cheese pizza, thin crust‡	1/4 of a 15-oz size pizza or a 10" pizza	1 medium-fat meat, 2 starches, 1 fat
Chili with beans†‡ (commercial)	1 cup (8 oz)	2 medium-fat meat, 2 starches, 2 fats
Chow mein (without noodles or rice)†‡	2 cups (16 oz)	2 lean meat, 1 starch, 2 vegetable
Macaroni and cheese‡	1 cup (8 oz)	1 medium-fat meat, 2 starches, 2 fats

Soup

Food	Amount	Exchanges
Bean†‡	1 cup (8 oz)	1 lean meat, 1 starch, 1 vegetable
Chunky, all varieties‡	10 3/4-oz can	1 medium-fat meat, 1 starch, 1 vegetable
Cream (made with water)‡	1 cup (8 oz)	1 starch, 1 fat
Vegetable or broth‡	1 cup (8 oz)	1 starch
Spaghetti and meatballs‡ (canned)	1 cup (8 oz)	1 medium-fat meat, 1 fat, 2 starches
Sugar-free pudding (made with skim milk)	1/2 cup	1 starch

If beans are used as a meat substitute:

Food	Amount	Exchanges
Dried beans†, peas†, lentils†	1 cup (cooked)	1 lean meat, 2 starches

Foods for Occasional Use

Food	Amount	Exchanges
Angel-food cake	1/12 cake	2 starches
Cake, no icing	1/12 cake (3-in. square)	2 starches, 2 fats
Cookies	2 small (1 3/4 in. diameter)	2 starches, 1 fat
Frozen fruit yogurt	1/3 cup	1 starch
Gingersnaps	3	1 starch
Granola	1/4 cup	1 starch, 1 fat
Granola bars	1 small	1 starch, 1 fat
Ice cream, any flavor	1/2 cup	1 starch, 2 fats
Ice milk, any flavor	1/2 cup	1 starch, 1 fat
Sherbet, any flavor	1/4 cup	1 starch
Snack chips, all varieties‡	1 oz	1 starch, 2 fats
Vanilla wafers	6 small	1 starch, 2 fats

Starch Group	Uncooked	Cooked
Cream of Wheat	2 level tbsp	1/2 cup
Dried beans	3 tbsp	1/3 cup
Dried peas	3 tbsp	1/3 cup
Grits	3 level tbsp	1/2 cup
Lentils	2 tbsp	1/3 cup
Macaroni	1/4 cup	1/2 cup
Noodles	1/3 cup	1/2 cup
Oatmeal	3 level tbsp	1/2 cup
Rice	2 level tbsp	1/3 cup
Spaghetti	1/4 cup	1/2 cup

Meat Group		
Chicken	1 small drumstick	1 oz
	1/2 of a whole chicken breast	3 oz
Hamburger	4 oz	3 oz

† = 3 grams or more of fiber per serving.
‡ = 400mg or more of sodium per serving.

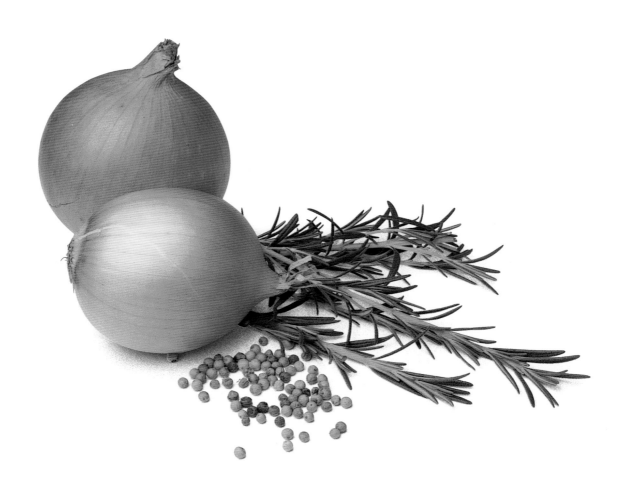

Index

Italics indicate photographs.